The
Natural
PHARMACIST

D0720308

Inside—Find the Answers to These Questions and More

☑ Can echinacea reduce my cold and flu symptoms? (See page 61.)

☑ Will it help me get over a cold and flu faster? (See page 55.)

☑ What's the proper dose of echinacea? (See page 74.)

☑ Which type of echinacea should I use? (See page 5.)

☑ Are there any side effects? (See page 91.)

☑ Why is echinacea not the best choice for preventing colds? (See page 63.)

☑ Can ginseng help prevent colds? (See page 105.)

☑ Can vitamin E improve immunity? (See page 129.)

☑ Can andrographis reduce cold symptoms? (See page 111.)

☑ What form of zinc should be used for colds? (See page 126.)

THE NATURAL PHARMACIST Library

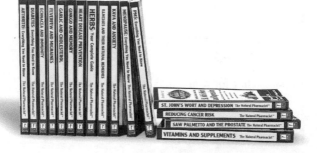

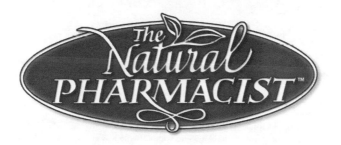

Everything You Need to Know About

Echinacea and Immunity

Elizabeth W. Collins, N.D.
Nancy Berkoff, R.D., Ed.D.

Series Editors
Steven Bratman, M.D.
David Kroll, Ph.D.

A DIVISION OF PRIMA PUBLISHING

Visit us online at www.thenaturalpharmacist.com

Warning—Disclaimer

This book is not intended to provide medical advice and is sold with the understanding that the publisher and the authors are not liable for the misconception or misuse of information provided. The authors and Prima Publishing shall have neither liability nor responsibility to any person or entity with respect to any loss, damage, or injury caused or alleged to be caused directly or indirectly by the information contained in this book or the use of any products mentioned. Readers should not use any of the products discussed in this book without the advice of a medical professional.

The Food and Drug Administration has not approved the use of any of the natural treatments discussed in this book. This book, and the information contained herein, has not been approved by the Food and Drug Administration.

Pseudonyms have been used throughout to protect the privacy of the individuals involved

PRIMA HEALTH and colophon are trademarks of Prima Communications, Inc.
THE NATURAL PHARMACIST is a trademark of Prima Communications, Inc.

Illustrations by Helene D. Stevens. Illustrations © 1999 Prima Publishing. All rights reserved.

All products mentioned in this book are trademarks of their respective companies.

Library of Congress Cataloging-in-Publication Data

Collins, Elizabeth W., N.D.
    Echinacea and immunity / Elizabeth W. Collins, Nancy Berkoff.
        p.   cm. — (The natural pharmacist)
    Includes bibliographical references and index.
    ISBN 0-7615-1558-5
    1. Echinacea (Plant)—Therapeutic use.   2. Immunological adjuvants.
3. Natural immunity.   I. Berkoff, Nancy.   II. Title.
RM165.E4C64 1999
615'.32399—dc21   98-43578
                                                                              CIP

00 01 02 HH 10 9 8 7 6 5 4 3 2
Printed in the United States of America

Visit us online at www.thenaturalpharmacist.com

Contents

What Makes This Book Different?

The interest in natural medicine has never been greater. According to the National Association of Chain Drug Stores, 65 million Americans are using natural supplements, and the number is growing! Yet it is hard for the consumer to find trustworthy sources for balanced information about this emerging field. Why? Frankly, natural medicine has had a checkered history. From snake oil potions sold at the turn of the century to those books, magazines, and product catalogs that hype miracle cures today, this is a field where exaggerated claims have been the norm. Proponents of natural medicine have tended to abuse science, treating it more as a marketing tool than a means of discovering the truth.

But there is truth to be found. Studies of vitamins, minerals, and other food supplements have been with us since these nutritional substances were first discovered, and the level and quality of this science has grown dramatically in the last 20 years. Herbal medicine has been neglected in the United States, but in Europe, this, the oldest of all healing arts, has been the subject of tremendous and ongoing scientific interest.

At present, for a number of herbs and supplements, it is possible to give reasonably scientific answers to the questions: How well does this work? How safe is it? What types of conditions is it best used for?

THE NATURAL PHARMACIST series is designed to cut through the hype and tell you what we know and what we don't know about popular natural treatments. These books are more conservative than any others available, more honest about the weaknesses of natural approaches, more fair in their comparisons of natural and conventional treatments. You won't find any miracle cures here, but you will discover useful options that can help you become healthier.

Why Choose Natural Treatments?

Although the science behind natural medicine continues to grow, this is still a much less scientifically validated field than conventional medicine. You might ask, "Why should I resort to an herb that is only partly proven, when I could take a drug with solid science behind it?" There are at least three good reasons to consider natural alternatives.

First, some herbs and supplements offer benefits that are not matched by any conventional drug. Vitamin E is a good example. It appears to help prevent prostate cancer, a benefit that no standard medication can claim. Also, vitamin E almost certainly helps prevent heart disease. While there are standard drugs that also prevent heart disease, vitamin E works differently and may be able to complement many of the other approaches.

Another example is the herb milk thistle. Studies strongly suggest that this herb can protect the liver from injury. There is no pill or tablet your doctor can prescribe to do the same.

Even if the science behind some of these treatments is less than perfect, when the risks are low and the possible benefit high, a treatment may be worth trying. It is a little-known fact that for many conventional treatments the science is less than perfect as well, and physicians must balance uncertain benefits against incompletely understood risks.

A second reason to consider natural therapies is that some may offer benefits comparable to those of drugs with fewer side effects. The herb St. John's wort is a good example. Reasonably strong scientific evidence suggests that this herb is an effective treatment for mild to moderate depression, while producing fewer side effects on average than conventional medications. Saw palmetto for benign enlargement of the prostate, ginkgo for relieving symptoms and perhaps slowing the progression of Alzheimer's disease, and glucosamine for osteoarthritis are other examples. This is not to say that herbs and supplements are completely harmless—they're not—but for most the level of risk is quite low.

Finally, there is a philosophical point to consider. For many people, it "feels" better to use a treatment that comes from nature instead of from a laboratory. Just as you might rather wear all-cotton clothing than polyester, or look at a mountain landscape rather than the skyscrapers of a downtown city, natural treatments may simply feel more compatible with your view of life. We can quibble endlessly about just what "natural" means and whether a certain treatment is "actually" natural or not, but such arguments are beside the point. The difference is in the feeling, and feelings matter. In fact, having a good feeling about taking an herb may lead you to use it more consistently than you would a prescription drug

Of course, at times synthetic drugs may be necessary and even lifesaving. But on many other occasions it may be quite reasonable to turn to an herb or supplement instead of a drug.

To make good decisions you need good information. Unfortunately, while hundreds of books on alternative medicine are published every year, many are highly misleading. The phrase "studies prove" is often used when the studies in question are so small or so badly conducted that they prove nothing at all. You may even find that the "data" from other books come from studies with petri dishes and not real people!

You can't even assume that books written by well-known authors are scientifically sound. Many of these authors rely on secondary writers, leading to a game of "telephone," where misconceptions are passed around from book to book. And there's a strong tendency to exaggerate the power of natural remedies, whitewashing them with selective reporting.

THE NATURAL PHARMACIST series gives you the balanced information you need to make informed decisions about your health needs. Setting a new, high standard of accuracy and objectivity, these books take a realistic look at the herbs and supplements you read about in the news. You will encounter both favorable and unfavorable studies in these pages and will learn about both the benefits and the risks of natural treatments.

THE NATURAL PHARMACIST series is the source you can trust.

Steven Bratman, M.D.
David Kroll, Ph.D.

Introduction

Colds and flus are among the most common illnesses in the world. You've probably suffered from your share. Most likely, you've experienced many days of lost productivity, not to mention a whole lot of misery. Although colds and flus are usually not very serious, they are easily transmitted from person to person. To compound matters, when people don't feel sick enough to stay home, they go out—to work, to the grocery store, to movies, and so on—and infect others because they think the cold "isn't that bad." For that reason, most people can count on getting a couple of colds and maybe one flu each year.

For some people, though, colds are almost constant companions through the winter. It can be difficult to tell when one ends and the next one begins. In these cases, a couple of factors usually contribute to the excessive number of colds. One factor is *exposure:* If you teach first grade, you are probably exposed to more colds and flus than someone who works in a small office. Another factor is *susceptibility:* Your immune system may be weakened by poor nutrition, stress, or other causes, making you a prime target for a cold or flu virus.

There are no good medical treatments for colds. Many medications are available to help you manage the symptoms so you can get on with your life, but they are in no way cures. You can get decongestants, cough medications, and lozenges to relieve your sore throat. You can choose from day and night preparations and different medications for adults and children. If you are lucky, you can use these medications without side effects like drowsiness and difficulty concentrating. Unfortunately, for many people, the treatment is not much better than the illness. You can go to work, but you can't focus; all you really want to do is take a nap.

For flu, we are somewhat better off. There is a vaccination to prevent it and two effective medications as well. However, these work only against certain specific forms of flu.

Another option for both colds and flus is the herb echinacea. This flower has been used medicinally for hundreds of years, initially by Native Americans and later by European settlers and travelers who brought the plant back to Europe. Echinacea is a very popular herb in Germany, prescribed by many physicians as the primary treatment for colds and flus. It is used alone and in combination with other herbs and also in combination with antibiotics when they are deemed appropriate.

Among the medicinal herbs used in the United States, echinacea is one of the most popular. Double-blind studies suggest that—while not a cure for the common cold—echinacea can help you get over your cold faster and reduce the symptoms while you are sick. It may also sometimes "abort" a cold if taken at the beginning of symptoms. However, the evidence suggests that taking echinacea regularly throughout the cold season will not significantly reduce the number of colds you will develop.

If you're curious about natural medicine and are looking for an easy place to start your exploration, echinacea may provide an excellent introduction. It's easy to find, commonly used, and low in side effects. Also, you don't have to make any hard decisions. Sometimes when you think about using alternative treatments, you have to make serious choices about whether to use conventional medications in order to avoid harm. For colds, however, there is no effective conventional medication, so you have little to lose by experimenting with echinacea. In this book, we'll explain what the research tells us about this useful flower, and we'll tell you how to buy it and use it. We'll also discuss other popular natural cold remedies, giving you information to make the most educated choice you can.

CHAPTER

ONE

What Is
Echinacea?

Echinacea (pronounced "ek-ih-NAY-sha") is a native North American plant that grows wild and in gardens throughout the United States. A member of the aster (or *Compositae*) family, it is related to the asters you may have in your garden. Each flower head has a large, dark central cone surrounded by daisy-like petals that may be purple, white, yellow, coral, or red, depending on the species (see figure 1). The echinacea plant is generally stiff and grows upright in dense clusters as high as 5 feet tall.[1]

The common name most often used for echinacea is "purple coneflower," which refers to the most common leaf color in current cultivation and the striking central cone of the flower head. Many of the other names people have used for echinacea over the years describe where the plant was grown or how it was traditionally used. For example, your grandmother may have known the plant as either Missouri snakeroot or Kansas snakeroot because it grows wild in both states and was used by Native

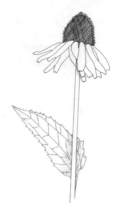

Figure 1. *Echinacea purpurea,* also known as purple coneflower

Americans to heal snake bites. Despite its many descriptive names, most North Americans simply call the plant by its Latin name: *echinacea.*

The word *echinacea* comes from the Greek word "echinos," which means sea urchin or hedgehog. It probably got this name from the prickly spikes found on the flower head. Eight species of echinacea have been identified, but only three are commonly used as medicinal herbs: *E. purpurea, E. angustifolia,* and *E. pallida.*

Echinacea, like many medicinal plants, is a weed that has become popular with gardeners. It is easy to grow from seed, will grow in drought conditions, and even adapts to rocky soil. At the end of its growing season, echinacea produces lots of seeds that will give you an even denser patch of beautiful

Echinacea has become popular with gardeners; it's easy to grow, is hearty, and adapts well to rocky soil.

coneflowers the following year. You can also cultivate echinacea as a perennial by trimming the stalks to a few inches above the ground and letting the plants grow back the following year.

What Is in Echinacea?

While scientists have identified many chemicals found in some or all the echinacea species, few researchers agree on which chemicals are the active medicinal components. Still, the vast quantity of research has given us a good idea of what chemicals echinacea contains, as well as ideas about what these chemicals do.

Echinacea contains several components that produce varying effects both in animals (including humans) and in cell populations in test tubes. Some components are found in the roots; some exist only in the flowers or stems. Some are

Double-blind studies give us evidence that all three types of echinacea do indeed work.

water-soluble and some alcohol-soluble, which is important information when you make or buy medicinal extracts of echinacea. Not all constituents are found in every variety of echinacea, though some are common to several. Because the chemical makeup of each species is different, it is difficult to say "this is the one chemical that makes echinacea work." Regardless, double-blind studies give us evidence that all three types of echinacea do indeed work.

Some of echinacea's known components are words you're probably not familiar with: caffeic acids, such as cichoric acid, echinacoside, caffaric acid, and cynarine;

flavonoids; immunostimulatory polysaccharides; polyacetylenes; alkylamides; isobutylamides; alkaloids; and essential oils.[2–5] Researchers have studied many of these
components in an attempt to understand what makes
echinacea work. Some of these studies will be explained in
chapter 5.

What Is the Difference Between the Types of Echinacea?

The three medicinal species of echinacea—*Echinacea angustifolia*, *Echinacea purpurea*, and *Echinacea pallida*—
are similar but not identical. Researchers have studied
various species, sometimes alone and sometimes in combination, but it is not clear which variety is most effective.
There are, though, definite chemical differences among
the three medicinal types of echinacea. All three have different combinations and amounts of the components listed
above, which gives each species its own chemical fingerprint.

Echinacea angustifolia

The *angustifolia* species of echinacea can grow up to 1 to
2 feet tall. It has narrow leaves and deep purple flowers
that bloom from May through August. This species, which
likes dry, rocky areas, grows from Minnesota to Texas and
in Colorado and Montana.[6] Because this variety is not easily cultivated, much of the *E. angustifolia* sold is harvested
from the wild.

The Native Americans in the plains region used *E. angustifolia* more than any other medicinal plant.[7] Because
of this, Europeans who settled in North America were
most familiar with this variety, so European herbal product manufacturers originally concentrated on acquiring *E.
angustifolia*. During a period when American sources did
not meet the European demand, Dr. Gerhard Madaus,

president of Madaus and Company, a German pharmaceutical firm, went to the United States on an echinacea seed–procurement trip. Hoping that his company might be able to successfully grow its own crop in Germany, Dr. Madaus purchased what he thought were *E. angustifolia* seeds but that were, in fact, seeds of *E. purpurea*. Madaus and Company successfully cultivated *E. purpurea* and manufactured products using the herb. This case of mistaken identity is the primary reason *E. purpurea* has become the

E. purpurea is the most prevalent variety of echinacea in current medical use.

main type of echinacea we use today, though some herbalists still believe that *E. angustifolia* is preferable medicinally. One study suggests that *E. angustifolia* taken daily at the beginning of cold season can slightly reduce the incidence of colds in people especially susceptible to them (see chapter 5). However, *E. angustifolia* does not seem to reduce the incidence of colds in healthy people.

Echinacea purpurea

The tallest echinacea species, *E. purpurea* is characterized by flowers ranging from pale purple to dark purple and petals that may be tipped with yellow. Its lower leaves look as if they have small teeth on them, distinguishing this type from the other two common medicinal varieties. *E. purpurea* is the most prevalent variety of echinacea in current medical use (as explained above). The species grows in the open woods or prairies from Virginia to Georgia and Louisiana, west to Texas, and north to Ohio, Illinois, and Michigan, flowering from June through October.[8]

E. purpurea root contains more cichoric acid than either *E. angustifolia* or *E. pallida* (actually, *E. pallida* doesn't contain any of this acid).[9-12] Most *E. purpurea* preparations are made from the leaves and flowers, although the root is also used. A recent study suggests that *E. purpurea* can "abort" a cold if taken at the onset of symptoms, and in earlier studies it was found to reduce the duration and severity of cold symptoms (see chapter 5). As with *E. angustifolia,* regular use of *E. purpurea* does not seem to reduce the incidence of colds in healthy people.

Echinacea pallida

E. pallida is the shortest of the echinacea plants, growing only about 18 inches high. It has long leaves that tend to droop and flowers that range in color from rose to white. This species likes rocky areas and woods and grows well from northeast Texas to southwest Wisconsin, where it blooms in June and July.[13]

The roots of *E. pallida,* which Native Americans used for infectious diseases and snake bites, are the part most often used today. The dense roots of *E. pallida* are easy to harvest and may have provided the bulk of the echinacea root used in North America for many years, although many suppliers claimed it was *E. angustifolia.*[14]

E. pallida's chemical components are not dramatically different from those of *E. purpurea,* except that *E. pallida* does not contain cichoric acid.[15-18] Another interesting note is that *E. pallida* does not contain a significant quantity of alkylamides. These components of liquid echinacea preparations are what make your tongue tingle after you take them; their absence in *E. pallida* means that the variety does not produce a tingling sensation.[19]

Whether or not the presence of alkylamides makes a difference medicinally is unclear; however, their presence is certainly noticeable when you take most liquid echinacea. Some herbalists tell you to watch for the characteristic tingling to ensure that you have good-quality echinacea. While it may not be accurate as a signal of quality, tingling definitely helps you identify species. If you've purchased a liquid identified as *E. angustifolia* or *E. purpurea* and your tongue doesn't tingle when you take it, you have either *E. pallida* or something that isn't echinacea at all.

A recent study found that *E. pallida* can reduce the duration of colds and flus (see chapter 5).

What Was Echinacea Used for Historically?

Native Americans have used echinacea medicinally for perhaps thousands of years, long before they introduced it to European settlers early in the nineteenth century. The herb was soon widely used among Europeans as well. At that time, many people practiced some form of herbal medicine on their own, rather than seeing the doctors of the day, who often used medical techniques such as bloodletting, leeching, purging, and prescribing ingestion of toxic heavy metals. The colonists brought many common household herbs from Europe and grew them alongside native North American plants in herb gardens to provide much of the medicine they used in daily life.

In some Native American tribes, echinacea was considered the king of medicines. They made juice or tea from the fresh flower, pulp from the roots, and even smoke from dried echinacea flowers to help many of their common ailments.

One of the first written mentions of the medicinal use of echinacea was made by Constantine Rafinesque, a self-taught botanist and founder of the "Eclectic" school of medical thought. The Eclectics were physicians who

Echinacea Use by Native Americans

Native American tribes often used echinacea for medicinal purposes, such as those listed below, showing the high esteem this medicinal herb earned among Native American healers.

- toothache, sore neck, burns, headache, menstrual cramps
- inflammation of the eyes, gums, mouth, throat, joints
- abdominal problems and indigestion
- fever
- snakebites and other poisonous bites and stings
- cough and colds, tonsillitis
- infectious diseases: mumps, measles, smallpox
- gonorrhea

Adapted from Paul Bergner, *The Healing Power of Echinacea and Goldenseal* (Prima, 1997)

believed in using any method or medicine that might be useful in improving health. Great proponents of botanical medicines, the Eclectics wrote books detailing the medicinal uses of many Western plants.[20]

Rafinesque traveled widely, studying and recording the uses of North American plants. He studied with many Native American tribes to learn how they used the plants in their native areas before the tribes were resettled onto reservations. Rafinesque recorded a wealth of knowledge about North American medicinal plants. His *Medical Flora* (1831) was a major text in medical schools for over 80 years.

The popularity of echinacea owes much to the Eclectics, as they advocated its use. Rafinesque initially described echinacea's use, and the influential Eclectic physician Dr. John King elaborated on it in the first Eclectic *materia medica* (a reference listing medicinal plants and homeopathic remedies) in 1852. During the next 50 years, the Eclectics established uses for and created preparations of echinacea.

In the late 1800s, echinacea became wildly popular because of a Dr. H.C.F. Meyer (whose professional training and background has been described in many ways, from simply unknown to distinctly questionable). Dr. Meyer traveled the country during the 1880s and 1890s selling an herbal concoction containing echinacea, among other ingredients. This mixture was proclaimed (at least by Dr. Meyer) to cure at least 30 diseases and conditions, including skin diseases, snake bites, headaches, malaria, cholera, typhoid, and blood poisoning.

Dr. Meyer promoted his formula with great verve, using techniques reminiscent of religious revival movements. He was even reputed to have volunteered to be bitten by a rattlesnake and subsequently cured with echinacea to prove the herb's potency. He promoted echinacea to the Lloyd Brothers Pharmacy (a firm that prepared over 300 herbal remedies from North American medicinal plants) and to Eclectic physicians, many of

In the late 1800s, echinacea became wildly popular in America.

whom were at least initially skeptical. Ultimately, though, whether or not they believed in the efficacy of Dr. Meyer's herbal remedy, the Eclectics and the Lloyd Brothers were certainly convinced of echinacea's value.

Despite its dubious reputation as a "snake oil" remedy (thanks to Dr. Meyer), echinacea was eventually used by

> **In Germany, echinacea is the most commonly prescribed treatment for the common cold.**

serious physicians. By the 1920s, the Lloyd Brothers Pharmacy reported that echinacea was the best-selling product in the history of their company. Echinacea continued to be a very popular cold and flu remedy in the United States until the development of sulfa antibiotics. Ironically, antibiotics are not at all effective for colds and flus, which are usually viral infections untouched by antibiotics, while echinacea *does* appear to be beneficial in such cases (see chapter 5).

Although physicians in the United States and Canada eventually stopped using herbal remedies in general, including echinacea, the herb didn't fall out of favor in Europe. A mounting body of scientific evidence led Germany, in 1992, to authorize the use of echinacea root extracts for "the supportive treatment of flu-like infec-

> **Echinacea is one of the most popular medicinal herbs in the United States today.**

tions" and echinacea juice for "supportive treatment of recurrent infections of the upper respiratory tract and lower urinary tract."[21] In Germany today, at least 300 products on the market contain echinacea, and the herb is the most commonly prescribed treatment for the common cold.

In the United States, however, patients request and physicians too frequently prescribe antibiotics for colds, despite the fact that antibiotics are ineffective against viruses.

Medical authorities frown on this widespread practice because it contributes to the development of "superbugs," bacteria resistant to all antibiotics. Luckily, echinacea may offer some protection against colds but does not contribute to the "superbug" problem. The public has begun to embrace echinacea: it has become one of the most popular medicinal herbs in the United States, with over $300 million in sales in 1995.

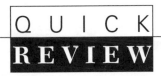

QUICK REVIEW

- Three species of echinacea are used medicinally: *E. purpurea, E. angustifolia,* and *E. pallida.* We have no evidence that one is better than another.
- Although considerable research has focused on discovering echinacea's components and active ingredients—and many have been identified—no single active ingredient has been isolated. In short, we don't know exactly what makes echinacea work.
- For centuries, Native Americans have used echinacea to treat a variety of ailments.
- Many European physicians use echinacea today, especially those in Germany, where the herb is presently an approved drug, used primarily for colds and flus.
- Echinacea is a commonly used herbal remedy in North America.

The Immune System Made Simple

Before we discuss how echinacea can help you fight colds and flus, you need to understand how your immune system works and what happens when you get sick. (If you want to skip right to a chapter about echinacea, turn to chapter 5 or 6.)

Many people like to think of their immune system as their own personal army, protecting their body from "foreign invaders." When you are exposed to any bacteria, virus, allergen, or other foreign substance, your immune system responds to this invasion without your having to think about it. The cells and chemicals of your immune system catch and immobilize invaders, making sure they can't infect you further. We have a beautiful, intricate, and very sophisticated system within our bodies.

The Basics of Immunity

We all know that the immune system fights the invaders that make us sick, but few of us understand how it knows what to get rid of. The body has an incredibly sophisticated system for recognizing foreign invaders, such as bacteria or viruses. These foreign objects are called antigens.

In response to antigens, some parts of your immune system simply perform a seek-and-destroy mission. Other parts orchestrate responses specific to each antigen that are carried out by yet *other* parts of the immune system— sort of like command central sitting back in the map room monitoring progress and telling the troops where to go and what to do. Over time, your immune system learns and adapts to become better at fighting specific antigens— enemies your body has encountered before.

The Nuts and Bolts of the Immune System

The most basic components of your immune system are the *white blood cells* (also known as *leukocytes,* which is Latin for "white cells"). They are manufactured in your bone marrow and lymphatic tissues (like the lymph nodes in your neck, which swell up when you have a sore throat). After they're made, these white blood cells move into your bloodstream; there, they can travel to the site of an infection quickly. Some white blood cells are always circulating in your body, but when you have an infection your body makes more to combat the infection more efficiently. It's like calling up the reserves during a war. They're trained and ready when you need them, and they must simply be summoned into action.

Over time, your immune system learns and adapts to become more efficient.

When you have an infection, your body starts to make more white blood cells within hours.

Your doctor can order a blood test called a *white blood cell count* to learn whether you have an increase of some types of white blood cells, which can indicate certain types of serious infection.

Your immune system has two general parts: *innate* and *learned*. The innate part reacts to everything in a general way, while the learned part reacts a bit differently for each antigen.

Innate Immunity

Innate immunity responds in the same way to everything it detects that is different from your cells. It's efficient, but it lacks finesse. Every antigen gets the same response, and every immune cell that's part of your innate immunity does the same job every time. In fact, the cells of the innate immune system respond the same way in all people. In addition to some types of white blood cells, other examples of innate immunity are your stomach acid and digestive enzymes, which break down most foreign substances they encounter.

Your innate immune system includes several types of white blood cells. Each different type does specific tasks, but they all work together to get rid of anything that isn't you. Two of the cell types that make up your innate immune system are *granulocytes* and *macrophages*.

Granulocytes are so named because these cells contain small granules of chemicals. These granules help the granulocytes destroy foreign substances they contact, usually ones that have been "tagged" by another part of the immune system. Basically, these cells will do one of two things when they find an antigen: either they envelop and digest it using their chemicals, or they spit the chemicals out at the antigen. Either way, the foreign thing is going to get broken down by the chemicals.

Immune System Glossary

acquired immunity. Also known as learned immunity. Results from exposure to foreign substances that your body learns to recognize and respond to.

antibody. Antigen-fighting substance made by B-lymphocytes in response to exposure to a specific antigen. Helps destroy antigens.

antigen. A foreign substance that causes the body to produce antibodies.

B-lymphocyte. A type of white blood cell that produces antibodies specific to the antigen that stimulated the antibody production.

granulocyte. A white blood cell that contains granules of chemicals that can, on contact, kill microorganisms.

innate immunity. Also known as natural immunity. Immunity that is present at birth and does not require the immune system to recognize and adapt to specific antigens.

leukocyte. White blood cell.

lymphocyte. A type of white blood cell that is the main component in acquired immunity.

When these cells pull an antigen inside themselves, it's called *phagocytosis* (see figure 2). The more they can do this, the faster they'll get rid of the antigens. This is important to remember when we discuss the research on echinacea. Some of these granulocytes travel in your

macrophage. A cell of the innate immune system whose function is to recognize and ingest foreign substances.

NK cells. Specialized cells (also known as natural killer cells) that kill your own cells when your cells have become infected or are malfunctioning.

phagocytosis. The process of ingestion and destruction of a substance by a cell such as a granulocyte.

t-cells. Cells that directly attack virus-infected and foreign cells in a highly specific way, as well as coordinate other aspects of immunity.

white blood cell. Also called leukocyte. General term for a number of cells (including granulocytes, monocytes, and t-cells) that act to protect against infections. Some destroy antigens, some trigger others to destroy antigens, and some clean up the fragments left over after an antigen has been destroyed.

white blood cell count. A blood test that can identify the number of white blood cells present in a person's circulation and can differentiate the types of cells.

blood, waiting to be pulled into tissue where an infection is raging.

Other white blood cells, called *macrophages*, actually spend most of their time within your tissues waiting to gobble up ("phagocytize") invaders. Another task these

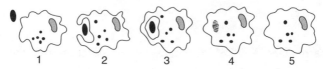

Figure 2. *A granulocyte ingesting and destroying an antigen*

specific cells perform, once they've started to digest the antigens, is to show them to other cells called *t-cells*. T-cells are very important, as they are part of the link between innate and learned immunity. Echinacea may enhance the t-cells' ability to do their jobs.

Camouflaged Invaders

One final important type of innate immune cell is the *natural killer*, or NK, cell. These specialized cells kill your own cells when the cells have become infected or are malfunctioning.

How do your own cells become the problem? Viruses often reproduce inside your own cells, hiding from your immune system. If the virus is entirely inside your cells, your immune system may just recognize the cell as you, not seeing the small changes that occur with viral infection. This lets the virus reproduce in very large numbers, so it can infect more cells.

NK cells are specialized to recognize these subtle changes in your cells, changes that cause them to look less like you but still not entirely foreign.

Acquired (or Learned) Immunity

In contrast to your innate immunity, you also have something called *acquired immunity*. This is the part of your immune system that *changes* as it is exposed to different substances, for example when you are immunized or when you are exposed to a cold or flu virus. This type of immunity does not use one-size-fits-all solutions, but rather has the sophistication of a fine European tailor. Every antigen gets a response that fits only itself, that is tailor-made (or lymphocyte-made) for it. Unlike your sense of taste, which can only distinguish between six different types of flavors, your immune system can "sense" literally millions of different kinds of antigens.

The cells of your acquired, or learned, immune system are called *lymphocytes*. There are many types of lymphocytes, each of which is patterned to recognize and help get rid of a specific antigen. Lymphocytes are made in the bone marrow and thymus and stored in the lymphatic organs like the spleen and lymph nodes.

The first time you contact a new antigen, some of your lymphocytes learn to recognize it, then they multiply and help kill the antigen. The next time you encounter that antigen, the lymphocytes that recognize it multiply even faster, enabling you to get rid of it more easily. You may

White blood cells, called *macrophages*, actually spend most of their time within your tissues waiting to gobble up ("phagocytize") invaders.

get sick the first time you encounter a particular antigen, but the next time you won't get so sick because your immune system will remember it be able to respond faster.

Lymphocytes work in many different ways. Some simply help "tag" antigens so that other cells will recognize and destroy them, while others produce chemicals that act as messengers between the cells of your immune system. Some even act to "turn off" the immune response once the antigen has been eliminated. In general, however, lymphocytes lead the attack.

Some specific types of lymphocytes are called B-lymphocytes and T-lymphocytes. The B-lymphocytes respond to the antigen by making substances called *antibodies*. Antibodies bind themselves to the antigen, making it impossible for the antigen to infect your other cells and tissues. It would be like having a huge board strapped to your back, then trying to fit through a doorway. You'd still be able to move (if you were strong), but you'd never fit through the door. You'd have to stay where you were. Once antibodies have grabbed the antigens, they just hold on and wait for other immune cells to come in for the kill.

You may get sick the first time you encounter a new antigen, but the next time you won't get so sick because your immune system will respond faster.

The B-lymphocytes make many copies of the antibodies, so they can immobilize many antigens. Each B-lymphocyte makes only one kind of antibody, though. It's like each B-lymphocyte has a pattern inside it and can make only antibodies that match that pattern. You have billions of different B-lymphocytes, one type for each antigen you have ever encountered. However, when you've been attacked by a certain antigen, your body creates a large reserve of the specific B-lymphocyte that can make antibodies against it. Should you be infected with the same antigen again, your body can rush these antibodies into production a lot faster than the first time.

Like antibodies, T-lymphocytes can bind directly to an antigen, and each T-lymphocyte is made for only one antigen. When you come in contact with an antigen, the T-lymphocytes that recognize it begin to reproduce very rapidly, making many identical T-lymphocytes. These identical cells, in turn, make other cells, called *activated t-cells*, that regulate your immune response. They are sort of like traffic cops, directing and making sure that everything gets to the right place in time. Activated t-cells make chemicals that affect other immune cells, stimulating them to do their jobs better.

Immune System Weakness Versus Immune Deficiency

In recent years, most of us have heard plenty of discussion about immune deficiency, especially in the context of AIDS (acquired immune deficiency syndrome) and leukemia. These are very serious medical conditions, in which entire sections of the immune system are severely disabled. Fortunately, tests are available that can detect and follow the progress of these illnesses, and, in many cases, excellent medical treatments are available for people who contract them. *Echinacea is not an appropriate treatment for these diseases.*

When we discuss immune system weakness in this book, we refer to something more subtle and less measurable than the serious sort of immune deficiency that is symptomatic of AIDS or leukemia. We refer to the condition of people who seem less able to fight off everyday infections like colds and flus, people who simply seem to get sick more often and for longer periods of time than they should, but without any good reason. You might call it "minor immune deficiency" as opposed to the "major immune deficiency" of AIDS and other conditions.

"Minor Immune System Weakness"

The title of this section isn't really a scientific term, but we're using it here to indicate the much more mild forms of immune weakness for which echinacea may be useful. Minor immune system weakness is not measurable through a white blood cell count. It's just that you catch colds too often and stay sick too long. In most cases, when people complain that their colds never seem to go away, doctors can find no abnormalities in their immune system. Whatever problem that might exist in the immune system is subtle. It's important to first make sure that no serious underlying medical condition or immunodeficiency exists. Then you might consider relatively simple causes for the repeated illness—such as excess stress, poor nutrition, and changes in your immune system that occur as you age.

Factors That Affect Immunity

As many factors affect your immune system as affect the rest of your body. Everything you eat or drink, where you live and work, your family history, existing medical conditions, travel, and everything else that makes up your daily life have an impact on your immune system.

Frequent colds and flus are not caused by an echinacea deficiency. Nor are they caused by a deficiency in cold medications, aspirin, acetaminophen, or anything else you may take in an effort to get better faster. You get colds and flus from a combination of your *susceptibility* and *exposure* to illnesses. If you are more susceptible when exposed to a communicable illness, you are more likely to get it than if you are exposed when you are less susceptible. There are many things that contribute to your level of susceptibility. You can control some, while others you cannot. Among those things you can control are your diet, stress level, sleep, exercise, and hygiene. Changes in all of

What you eat and drink, where you live, if you travel— all this and more affects your immune system.

these can and do affect your daily susceptibility to diseases like colds and flus (among others). By making choices that decrease your level of susceptibility, you improve your odds of successfully fighting off diseases. Still, some illnesses are strong enough to make you ill almost every time you come into contact with them (see chapter 3 for a further discussion of this concept). Sometimes you are so susceptible that even a weaker disease gets through and makes you sick.

If your immune system is functioning normally and you are healthy, you shouldn't get sick every time you come into contact with a communicable disease. If you get sick more than you think you should, look at your life and lifestyle to see whether any factors are present that might contribute to a weakened immune system. Among the most significant factors is stress.

Stress

Although stress is a vague and often misused term, it's an important factor in your health. A stressful event can be either negative or positive, physical or psychological. Major traumatic events such as having a sick relative, a death in the family, or financial troubles are certainly stressful. So are happy events such as getting married, buying a new home, retiring, or getting a promotion. Even much smaller things can be stressful, too—for example, not getting enough sleep on a regular basis, taking an exam, getting an annual physical, driving in bad traffic, and participating in strenuous exercise. Some of these events would be stressful to most people; others would be perceived as stressful by only some people.

What matters is more how you perceive and handle stress, rather than the specific event itself. If you perceive an event as stressful, it will cause the physical and emotional effects of stress in your body. On the other hand, if you perceive an event as manageable, it is less apt to produce stress effects. In addition, if you perceive an event as stressful but take steps to reduce the stress (talking to others, getting exercise, sleeping a little extra), your body will be able to manage the effects better than when you simply notice the stress and do nothing to reduce it.

You get colds and flus from a combination of your *susceptibility* and *exposure* to illnesses.

When you are under stress, your body reacts with the "fight or flight" response. This process causes the release of chemicals that increase your heart rate, breathing rate, blood pressure, and blood flow to your large muscle groups (such as those in your legs), as well as other responses. The net effect is that, when necessary, you can perform much more strenuous activities than you can under normal circumstances.

The fight or flight response comes in handy in emergencies—for instance, when you have to act fast to avoid a car accident. But our everyday stresses can cause our bodies to release these same chemicals. When you're constantly under stress, your body gets exhausted from producing these chemicals and having them overstimulate your body. You get run down, and nothing in your body works as well as it should.

When you're constantly under stress, your body gets exhausted from producing "fight or flight" chemicals.

Stress has many effects on the immune system. For instance, people under stress (including those undergoing medical procedures like surgery, as shown in one study) are more susceptible to infections than other people are.[1] Another study showed that reducing stress improves immunity in people fighting viral infections and even in people with cancer.[2]

While these studies don't suggest that stress reduction alone will cure you of disease, they suggest that stress may be one component of disease, and stress reduction may therefore be a component of getting better. Long-term or chronic stress is *not* harmless. Reduce the stress you can, so you can better cope with the stress you can't eliminate.

Aging

Other factors influence the strength of your immune system. One of them is aging. While aging is not, in and of itself, always a state of decline, some aspects of our health typically do decline as we age. Biological changes do take place as we age, and many of these start when we are in our thirties. Humans in their thirties are different than they were when in their teens, and they change even more by the time they reach their fifties. Change is inevitable.

According to one study, reducing stress improves immunity in people fighting viral infections and even in people with cancer.

While we don't understand the mechanisms or reasons for most of the changes that occur with age, we are becoming more familiar with the changes themselves. For instance, we know that a decrease in bone marrow occurs. Bone marrow makes all our blood cells, so the older we get, the less we can respond to the need for more white blood cells (or more red cells, for that matter). It doesn't mean we can't make them, just that we have less bone marrow to do the job for us.

Poor Nutrition

One additional factor that can affect the immune system is poor nutrition. People suffering from vitamin and mineral malnutrition often have more than their share of infections. You need to maintain adequate calories and nutrients for your body to function properly, including your immune system. (This topic is discussed more fully in chapter 9.)

The vitamins and minerals that are important to proper functioning and maintenance of the immune system are listed in table 1. Protein deficiency, like vitamin and mineral deficiencies, is immunosuppressive, and studies also show that deficiencies in other nutrients such as essential fatty acids can decrease your body's ability to react to antigens. Anorexics and bulimics often suffer from malnutrition and may experience immune deficiency as a result, especially because of deficiencies of protein,

Table 1. Vitamins and minerals needed for a healthy immune system

Vitamin or Mineral	RDA for Adults	Immune System Effects
Zinc[3]	12–15 mg	proper function of white blood cells, especially T-lymphocytes and macrophages
Vitamin A	4,000–5,000 IU	T- and B-lymphocyte responses to antigens; may help phagocytosis
B complex[4-7]	B_1 (thiamin): 1–1.5 mg B_2 (riboflavin): 1.2–1.8 mg B_5 (pantothenic acid): 4–7 mg B_6: 1.5–2.0 mg B_{12}: 2 mcg	proper antibody response to antigens
Vitamin E[8,9,10]	12–15 IU	lymphocyte production and function
Copper[11,12]	No RDA (safe and adequate range is 1.5–3 mg)	normal function of lymphocytes and the bacteria-killing abilities of granulocytes

vitamins, and minerals. Protein deficiency can also occur in people who are dieting or who restrict what they eat for other reasons. People who consume adequate calories may still fail to get enough protein, for example, vegetarians who fail to educate themselves on how to eat a healthful, balanced vegetarian diet.

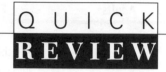

QUICK
REVIEW

- Your immune system is a complex and beautiful system. Its main job is to understand what is part of you and what is not part of you and to remove "antigens," the elements it perceives as not being part of you. In response to antigens, some parts of your immune system simply perform a seek-and-destroy mission (innate immunity). Other parts perform carefully orchestrated responses that are specific to each antigen (acquired immunity). Because your immune system can learn and adapt over time, it becomes more efficient.

- You get colds and flus from a combination of your *susceptibility* and *exposure* to illnesses.

- Many conditions can decrease your immunity. Factors that can have a negative effect on an otherwise healthy person's immune system are stress, aging, and poor nutrition.

Why Some People Get Infections Easily

You probably know someone who seems to get more than her share of the colds and flus going around, the person who always carries tissues and knows where every 24-hour pharmacy is in town. It may even be you. Although it is not unusual to have one or two colds per year, some of us seem to have more than our share.

While nothing is going to stop you from getting colds and flus entirely, there are things you can do to improve your odds. Knowing what causes colds, and how they are passed from your friends to you, can help. Taking steps to improve your general health also makes a difference. When you can't avoid a cold or flu, echinacea may help you feel better faster. As we shall see in chapter 5, echinacea may also be able to "ward off" some colds when it's taken early enough. However, regular use of echinacea does not seem to reduce the incidence of colds significantly.

Invisible but Powerful

What we know as the common cold is caused by many different viruses. There are more than 100 varieties of "rhinoviruses," the largest group of cold-causing viruses, just to give you one example. Medical books describe the common cold as an acute, self-limiting infection of the upper respiratory tract. If you think about it, you know what that means: sore throat, sneezing, headache, congestion, runny nose, and fatigue—all of which will eventually go away one way or another. Echinacea may be able to reduce these symptoms.

Facts About the Flu

In addition to the viruses that cause colds, there are influenza viruses that cause "flu." Influenza viruses come in three main classifications: type A, type B, and type C. Of the three, type A is by far the most common as well as the most potentially severe; type B is the second most common; and type C is relatively uncommon. The influenza A virus spontaneously changes a little from year to year, which is why you need a new vaccination every year. When it changes a great deal during a particular year, there is a more severe epidemic, because people's natural resistance developed from last year's flu doesn't protect them. Occasionally major changes occur, at which time we experience worldwide super-epidemics called pandemics, which can kill millions of people.

You can take steps to help prevent a cold.

Most years, the flu arrives in the late fall or early winter. The symptoms of influenza are similar to, though almost always more severe than, those of the common cold. The onset is usually sudden, with fever up to

103°F (39°C), severe exhaustion, and muscle and joint aches (especially in the back and legs) in addition to a prominent headache, runny nose, sore throat, and possibly a cough. As the illness pro-gresses, the muscle aches tend to get worse and the cough be-comes more prominent. You may notice that you're sensitive to light, your eyes may water, and you may even experience nausea and vomiting. While the majority of these symptoms should abate in a few days to a week, you may find that your fatigue and weakness linger and that you tend to sweat easily for weeks. Echinacea may be able to reduce some of these symptoms and reduce the time it takes to get better.

Echinacea may be able to reduce some flu symptoms and reduce the time it takes to get better.

People at High Risk for Flu Complications

Influenza can be dangerous for the very young and very old, women in the third trimester of pregnancy, and for those with lung disease, heart disease, kidney disease, diabetes, blood diseases (such as sickle-cell anemia), or immunosup-pression (as with AIDS or leukemia). Echinacea is not adequate treatment for people in these high-risk groups.

Flu can worsen chronic respiratory illnesses (like asthma and bronchitis), possibly leading to a need for hospitalization. Sometimes, flu can cause its own form of pneumonia, which usually requires hospitalization. Rare complications of flu include but are not limited to encephalitis (inflammation of the brain), myocarditis and pericarditis (inflammations of the heart), and Guillain-Barré syndrome.

A Clove of Garlic, a Bowl of Soup, and Thou

Completely unscientific folklore "cures" for the common cold have existed ever since groups of people have been living together. All across the world, caring for a cold seems to incorporate the same ideas: get lots of rest, drink plenty of fluids, stay warm, and eat healthful foods. The variations on this theme are very interesting (and sometimes scary or humorous). Here's what we found in sources from around the world.

Mexico: chicken broth laced with chilies (to make the victim sweat) and prayer

Lebanon: chicken or beef soup, no dairy products, alternating between sweating and being cool

Tibet: "soothing" foods (light in color, cooked slowly), tea with honey, avoiding spices

Israel: chicken soup, fruit and fruit juice, plenty of rest, staying away from other people

Why Me?

The viruses that cause colds and flus are easily spread from person to person, which might prompt you to ask why you always get sick while your best friend cruises through the year with a single cold that doesn't even slow him down. That's a difficult question to answer, as the reason one person gets sick while another doesn't involves so many variables. Part of the answer is exposure, but since most of us are exposed to these viruses frequently,

Poland: chicken and cabbage soup, mustard plaster (applied to chest), wearing garlic

Russia: chicken soup, herb teas; coarse salt wrapped in flannel, heated in the oven, and then applied to "sore" ears (the heat and salt were thought to "draw out" infection)

Korea: protein-rich soup, lots of steam (to "loosen up" the chest)

Norway: cod liver oil, boiled cod soup, sauna, mentholated rubs

Ireland: broth, wearing camphor sachet, daily prayer, keeping very warm

Ethiopia: thick porridge (rice or grain gruel), herb teas, smoking medicinal herbs

Italy: chicken broth with spinach or other greens, diluted wine (to "build the blood"), wearing garlic

Hungary: chicken or veal broth with egg noodles; a "tea" of mustard, vinegar, and garlic; black tea with lemon and sugar

that can't be the whole picture. Hygiene plays a role: Do you wash your hands frequently, especially after close contact with someone who has the flu? Finally, you would have to consider the more complicated issues of susceptibility and immune system, which we discussed in chapter 2.

Some diseases are very strong, and will make almost anyone exposed to them sick. Rabies is a good example. When a rabid animal bites, even the healthiest person is likely to come down with rabies. The best way to prevent this disease is to avoid exposure to rabid animals (a vaccine is also available).

How often you catch colds and flus depends mostly on your own immune strength.

Colds and flus, however, are more like opportunists, waiting for a weakened immune system to come along. The viruses are so common that most people are exposed to them many times every year. How often you get sick depends mostly on your own immune strength. Some years you may get sick once; other years you feel sick off and on most of the winter.

There are no conventional medications you can take to strengthen or stimulate your immune system. Vaccinations work—very specifically—to help you fight off certain illnesses, and they can help some with the flu, as we said above. In the case of the common cold, however, vaccinations are simply too specific to help with the hundreds of viruses that cause colds.

Echinacea may be able to improve the immune response to colds and flus in general. Other treatments such as vitamin E and ginseng may also be helpful, as described in chapters 8 and 9.

Over and Over Again

A young couple once came to me complaining that the good health both once enjoyed had deteriorated dramatically. Alex and Sarah reported that they had previously gotten no more than a couple of colds a year between them—until they had a child. During the first winter after Kyle's birth, both Sarah and Alex got sick slightly more often than usual. Then once their one-year-old went into daycare 2 days a week, they became really frustrated. Suddenly, they were sick as much as they were well, and both felt exhausted. Kyle got colds that barely slowed him down for a day or two, but Alex and Sarah really suffered. What had happened?

Most likely, many factors contributed. Both were sleeping less because they had a one-year-old, and they had less time to exercise, relax, and prepare healthful meals. This weakened their immunity. In addition, Kyle was in daycare, where he came into contact with lots of colds and flus, which he brought home to share. The combination of more exposure and weaker defenses meant a lot of colds.

To solve this problem, Alex and Sarah made a number of practical changes that I suggested. They took turns at child care so both partners could have some time to relax, even if that meant simply napping for an hour; they established a schedule so each could get enough sleep most of the time; and they took therapeutic doses of echinacea any time they felt they might be getting sick (dosage is discussed in chapter 6). After about 6 weeks, they reported only one cold each that slowed them down a little for a day or two. This was a big change for Sarah and Alex, and both were thrilled with the results.

Of course, a story like this does not prove the effectiveness of echinacea. I tell it to illustrate the common problem of frequent infections and to offer some steps sufferers can take to change the pattern. To discover whether echinacea itself is effective requires scientific research. In chapter 5, we will discuss scientific studies that suggest echinacea may indeed stimulate the immune system.

Factors You Can Control

What weakens the immune system? Physical and emotional stress, poor nutrition, and lack of exercise are a few basic factors. Remember the last time you had a cold? Did it by any chance correspond with a big deadline, family crisis, or even something less major but that kept you from sleeping well? People often report that they always seem to get sick just after they get home from a vacation or, worse, just as they leave for one. Add enough everyday stresses together, and you are likely to get sick.

Was Grandma Right About That Sweater?

According to folk tradition, getting chilled causes colds. Certainly people seem to catch more colds and flus when the weather turns wintry, but we don't know why. One theory holds that cold weather stimulates the flow of mucus, which may provide a good place for viruses to grow; but whether this situation actually contributes to the frequency of viral infections in humans is unknown. Another frequently stated explanation clearly has some truth to it: people tend to congregate more closely in the winter months, giving viruses a better opportunity to spread. You tend to be closer to other people all day long (who wants to eat lunch outside in the winter?) in a closed environment where others are sneezing and coughing. This situation helps transmit the viruses since more will remain floating in the air that you breathe in and you will spend more time breathing that air instead of outdoor air, in which viruses tend to disperse.

Add enough everyday stresses together, and you are likely to get sick.

Furthermore, you are likely to experience more physical shock from major temperature changes as you move between the cold outdoors and heated buildings. (The opposite happens in the summer, as you go from the outside heat into air-conditioned cars and buildings.) Exposure to sudden temperature changes may in some way weaken your immunity. Top it off with the stress of the holidays and the fact that you may be unable to get outside to practice your favorite form of exercise, and you may well get sick.

Stress

When you think of the word *stress*, do you picture yourself having a really bad day? As we discussed in chapter 2, stress can be anything, good or bad, that disrupts your sense of well-being. If you have good coping mechanisms and ways to decrease your stress level, stress won't have much of an effect on your immune system or the rest of your body. If you don't do things to decrease your stress levels, every system in your body works less efficiently.

Stress is defined in *Taber's* medical dictionary as when "a structure, system, or organism is acted upon by forces that disrupt equilibrium."[1] The definition goes on to say that biological systems need a certain amount of stress to maintain their well-being, but that too much stress can produce patho-

Prolonged intense exercise, such as running a marathon, is known to lower immunity.

logical changes. This makes a lot of sense. When you can maintain your equilibrium in the face of the stresses that keep your life interesting, you feel fine. When you experience so much stress that your personal coping mechanisms (perhaps sleep, exercise, hobbies, chocolate) can't

Betty's Story

Betty's story is a great example of how to catch a really bad cold. A retired bookkeeper, she was asked to cover some vacations in early December, and she was glad to earn the extra money for Christmas. Her grandkids were coming to visit for the last two weeks of December (and they were bringing their parents, too!). After working all day, Betty would go shopping and then spend her evening baking and preparing her house for her grandkids. For the first time since her kids were little, Betty was planning to "do Christmas right." Until December 23.

That day, Betty woke with a terrible sore throat and stuffy head. By the time she made it into my office in the afternoon, she had a low fever and a headache, and all she wanted to do was sleep. Mournfully, Betty asked why she had gotten sick *now.* She actually seemed surprised that it had happened, but when we talked about it, she realized that she had planned her

keep up, you get sick. There is no set stress level at which you will get sick; your tolerance for stress can change from week to week and year to year; and resistance to illness definitely varies from person to person.

You may think of stress only as psychological, but physical exertion is another form of stress. Extremely intense exercise, such as training for and running in a marathon, is known to lower immunity. Endurance athletes frequently get sick after maximal exertion. This is basically a "too much of a good thing" situation. Reasonable amounts of regular exercise (for example, half an hour three or four times per week) help decrease most people's perception of stress in their lives. When we exercise at a highly competitive level, or train intensely for a competi-

illness almost as well as she had planned her holiday. She'd worked in an office, being exposed to the recirculated air and lots of new people. She'd been in malls, again surrounded by new people (and their illnesses) much more than usual. She'd slept less. She'd eaten more than a few Christmas cookies and had cooked fewer nutritious meals.

Betty managed to get well enough to enjoy her holiday, but not without some sacrifices. She stopped preparing, realizing that she had done enough to make the holiday great, and she didn't want to make it more memorable by getting pneumonia and going to the hospital. She drank plenty of fluids and took echinacea, and by Christmas morning her cold was manageable. She wasn't quite up to peak performance, but she could at least enjoy her grandkids.

tive athletic event, we stress our bodies as we push them to perform. It isn't simply a matter of getting in better shape so your body can tolerate such training without being stressed; performance athletes will tell you that intense training is both exhilarating and stressful.

Nutrition

Your diet definitely affects your immune system, as well as the rest of your body. What you do (and do not) eat can make you more or less susceptible to illness. Eating well can help your immune system function optimally.

Make sure you're eating a balanced diet and getting enough vitamins and minerals, as well as adequate protein. If you are not well nourished, your body and your immune system can't function at their best. For a more complete discussion of this, see chapters 2 and 9.

Exercise and Sleep

Exercise and sleep help you live well. Regular, moderate exercise is like a reset button, clearing away the effects of stress and allowing your body to find its equilibrium. When you exercise regularly, you have better circulation of blood, better general health, more energy, and more restful sleep. In addition, as you become more fit, you'll find that you manage some tasks more easily.

Everyone knows the value of sleep, and most people (rightly) feel that they don't get enough. Sleep experts suggest most people function best on about 8 hours' sleep per night. A 20 to 30 minute nap, in addition to a good night's sleep, can go a long way toward keeping you healthy and feeling at your best. While you can do your job and live your life on too little sleep, you end up paying the price—fatigue, reduced alertness, and mood swings are classic signs of chronic sleep deprivation. Lack of sleep is definitely a stress. As we explained in chapter 2, too much stress weakens your immune system.

How Can Echinacea Help?

If, despite your efforts to ward off colds and flus, you get a cold or flu, echinacea can help. As we will explain in chapter 5, scientific studies have found that echinacea can lessen the severity and reduce the duration of colds and minor flus, especially if you start taking it early.

When to See a Doctor

It is important to note that colds and flus should not last too long or be too severe. These illnesses, as we said before, are generally self-limiting and not overly serious. You may be out of commission for a few days, but if you're sick more than a week, a trip to the doctor may be in order. You may not have just a cold or flu.

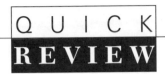

- Some people seem to get lots of colds and flus, while others are able to fight most of them off.

- Colds and minor flus are caused by a large number of viruses that conventional medicine has little ability to prevent or cure. (There are vaccines and treatments available that help prevent or minimize the effects of influenza type A.)

- Your immune system is your defense against the viruses that cause colds and flus. If your immune system is not working at its peak level, it may not be able to defend against the invading viruses, leaving you with a lot of colds or flus.

- Poor nutrition, emotional and physical stress, and lack of rest and exercise are some factors that can wear down your immune system, weakening its ability to respond to disease.

- If you get sick despite your best efforts (reducing stress, proper nutrition, adequate sleep and exercise), echinacea can lessen the severity and shorten the duration of colds and flus.

Conventional Treatments for Colds and Flus

I f you're like most people, you've probably spent your share of time in the cold and flu aisle of the pharmacy. Perhaps you read the labels, trying to weigh whether your sore throat or your stuffy head is the most prominent of your symptoms, and then decide to buy one of everything (and don't forget the extra box of tissues), just in case. These over-the-counter medications do help manage cold and flu symptoms once you have the illness, but that's about all they do. They won't rid your body of the virus that's making you sick or help your immune system get rid of the virus.

Some prescription medications can help prevent or shorten the duration of the flu if you take them early enough (we'll discuss these later in this chapter), but no medication as yet can help you avoid the common cold. Similarly, while you can get a shot to ward off some flus, no effective vaccine is available to prevent the common cold. Once a cold or flu is well established, the best advice your doctor will offer is that you should rest, drink lots of fluids, take acetaminophen for the headache, and wait for it to end. As long as your flu remains uncomplicated (you don't develop pneumonia, for example), this regimen will work well enough, though you aren't likely to enjoy it.

Wash, Wash, Wash Your Hands

It seems so basic, but proper hand washing is an important step in preventing colds and flus. We all know about washing our hands after we go to the bathroom or before and after handling food, but few of us think much about hand washing otherwise.

Colds and flus are spread through secretions from the mouth, throat, and nasal passages. These secretions can easily be passed from person to person, especially be-

Frequently washing your hands helps prevent cold viruses from being transferred from your hands to your eyes, mouth, or nose.

tween those in close contact. A sneeze or cough will spread the virus into the air or onto the hand or handkerchief of the person who sneezed or coughed. You might inhale the virus from the air, but you might also pick it up on your hands from a surface like a telephone recently touched by someone with the virus on their hands. If you take care of someone who has a cold or flu, you constantly touch surfaces on which the virus has settled. Although these viruses don't live for long outside the human body, they can survive long enough for

you to pick them up and transfer them to your own eyes, mouth, or nose. Frequently washing your hands helps pre-

And You Thought You Knew How to Wash Your Hands . . .

If your mom admonished you to wash both the front and back of your hands when you were a kid, she was right—but that is not enough. Many people wash their hands in under 10 seconds, and some never bother to use soap. A good hand washing takes 30 seconds and involves soap on all surfaces of the hands. You should lather thoroughly and rinse with your fingers down, so the water flows from your wrists to fingers. Finally, don't turn off the water (which you turned on with your dirty hands) with your newly clean hands. Get a paper towel from the dispenser, or get a tissue at home, and use that to touch the handle and turn off the water.

vent the viruses from taking advantage of the opportunity to invade your body.

If the bad news is that these viruses continually get onto your hands during cold and flu season, the good news is that your skin is a pretty good barrier. You don't get sick simply by touching someone who has a cold or flu or by touching something they have touched. You get sick when the virus actually makes contact with the mucous membranes that line your mouth and nose (your susceptibility, as described in chapters 2 and 3, is a factor as well). However, unconsciously wiping your nose or mouth can take the viruses right to their favorite point of entry.

The bottom line is that you need to wash your hands frequently, probably more than you normally do. You don't need to rush to the bathroom or to expensive "water-free" hand cleaners every time you touch something that someone else touched first. You do need to wash your hands before eating, before touching your mouth, eyes, or nose, and after being in close contact with someone who has a cold or flu. If you're taking care of someone who is infected, make sure she covers her mouth and nose when she sneezes or coughs, and wash your hands after you touch things she has handled, especially tissues or hand-kerchiefs, and every time you leave her room.

Using Vaccines to Prevent Flu

In chapter 2 we discussed immunity, one type of which was acquired immunity, also known as learned immunity. You get such immunity from being exposed to a virus or bacteria (or really any antigen) to which your body reacts by making antibodies and white blood cells specifically tai-lored to fight that single antigen. Some of these cells re-main in your body after you get well, and their presence speeds up your immune response the next time you en-counter the same antigen. You may not get sick at all on a repeat exposure and are unlikely ever to get as sick as you did the first time you encountered that antigen.

Immunizations, also known as vaccinations, work on this principle. Here's how vaccinations make you immune to diseases you've never caught: You are exposed (usually via injection) to a very small amount of an antigen, such as a weakened virus. Your body then mounts an immune re-sponse—producing antibodies and white blood cells spe-cific to this antigen. The next time you encounter that antigen, either through another immunization or "in the wild" (meaning from someone who is actually sick with the disease caused by the antigen—measles, for example), your immune system responds more quickly and effi-ciently, eliminating the antigen before you actually get

sick. This happens because the first exposure—the vaccination, for example—gives your immune system a head
start so you can quickly produce lots of antibodies and
lymphocytes to work against that antigen. Unfortunately, in the case of the com-
mon cold, no vaccine is available, primarily because so many
different viruses can cause a
cold. Vaccinating against every
virus that causes colds is simply
not possible.

**Up to 80% of
vaccinated indi-
viduals will man-
age to avoid the
flu entirely.**

For the flu, however, you
can protect yourself through a
relatively effective vaccine. Each
year, the flu vaccine is made
from the strain of flu that circu-
lated the year before. Assuming
the virus doesn't make a major shift, most people who get
the current vaccination before flu season rolls around will
get good protection. The quality of the protection varies,
depending on how similar the vaccine is to the virus circulating and the immune system status of the person exposed. If the vaccine closely matches the circulating virus,
up to 80% of vaccinated individuals will manage to avoid
the flu entirely.[1] Those who don't escape it entirely will
have many fewer complications and less severe cases of the
flu than unvaccinated people. Interestingly, the herb ginseng may augment the benefits of the flu vaccine (see
chapter 8).

This vaccine is not useful once you have the flu, but it
is a good preventive measure for those in groups at high
risk for exposing others (like health-care workers) or those
at risk for serious complications themselves (a list can be
found in chapter 3).

A new flu vaccine in the form of a nasal spray is just coming on the market at press time; it may be recommended for wide use among children to help stop the spread of the disease.

Antiviral Drugs for the Flu

Most people don't get the flu every year. If there isn't a major variation in the virus, your natural immunity to last year's flu (assuming you came down with it) may completely or partially protect you against this year's strain of flu. It is also possible that you may simply skate through the winter without being exposed. But what should you do if you didn't get vaccinated and someone who lives in the house with you gets sick? You may choose to use an antiviral medication to keep from getting a very bad case of the flu and to prevent the possible serious complications.

> **Amantadine and rimantadine are two drugs commonly used to diminish the severity of a flu, but you must take them early.**

Two drugs, amantadine and rimantadine, are commonly used to diminish the severity of a flu (technically, influenza A) once a person is exposed. These medications will only help if you take them within the first 48 hours after you develop symptoms. You can also take medication for prevention if you know you've been exposed. If someone in your house or at work has the flu, you could benefit by visiting your doctor early and asking about these medications. Also, your physician may provide a prescription for amantadine or rimantadine to have on hand at the beginning of flu season since they're relatively safe. Other medications that may be even more effective are working their way toward approval at press time.

Both rimantadine and amantadine can significantly decrease the duration and severity of flu symptoms. These medications appear to make it harder for a virus to multiply by interfering with a process called "uncoating" once the virus has entered your cells, one of the first steps in viral replication. This gives your immune system a chance to gear up before it must fight against untold trillions of the virus.

These medications are usually taken for a course of 10 days for treatment of an infection, or throughout the period of exposure for prevention. If you are sick and take one of these medications, you should rest and avoid exposing other people to your flu. You may not feel truly awful, but you still have the flu.

Echinacea appears to provide those suffering from colds with benefits similar to the benefits rimantadine and amantadine offer to flu sufferers.

Rimantadine is more commonly used than amantadine because it is equally effective and has fewer side effects. Amantadine is effective, but some people who take it (5 to 10%) have side effects such as anxiety, jitteriness, insomnia, and difficulty concentrating. These drugs are safe for most people, and they are generally effective in managing uncomplicated cases of the flu.

No equivalent drugs exist for the common cold. However, as we shall see in later chapters, echinacea appears to provide those suffering from either flu or a cold with benefits similar to the benefits rimantadine and amantadine offer to flu sufferers: milder symptoms and fewer days of illness. Please note that we do not know if echinacea provides the same benefits as standard medications in true influenza A.

The Pharmacy Shelf

Many over-the-counter medications are available for colds and flus. Most likely you've sampled them at some point with varying degrees of success. These medications can help with your symptoms to some extent, but they don't help you get better. The virus is still replicating in your cells, and you will need to wait until your immune system has things under control before you really feel like yourself again. Probably the most effective over-the-counter cold and flu treatments are the pain relievers and fever reducers, such as acetaminophen, aspirin, ibuprofen, and naproxen. They can significantly reduce the muscle aches and headache pain of the flu and may somewhat relieve the discomfort of a head cold.

The decongestants pseudoephedrine and phenyl-propanolamine may help relieve sinus discomfort, although they can also cause restlessness and insomnia and may increase blood pressure. They should not be used for more than four consecutive days because the body's adaptation to them can actually *cause* sinus congestion.

The expectorant guaifenesin, included in many cough syrups, can help break up thick mucus. Dextromethorphan is also a common ingredient in cough syrups. It suppresses a cough and is best used at night to help you sleep.

Antihistamines such as chlorpheniramine and tripolidine are often found in cold remedies, but neither is of much use in colds, except to help you fall asleep. Combination cold remedies contain many of these ingredients

Why Not Aspirin for a Child's Flu?

Aspirin is not found in cold and flu medications intended for children. This is because of the risks of Reye's syndrome. This illness, which was first recognized in the early 1960s, consists of encephalitis (swelling of the brain), nausea, vomiting, and liver damage. It occurs primarily in children under 18 years old. Reye's syndrome has been associated with the use of aspirin to treat an acute viral illness, like a flu, so unless directed by your pediatrician, you should never use aspirin for aches and fever in children. Acetaminophen and ibuprofen are just as effective and do not present this risk.

mixed together, often along with alcohol, but you will often do better by taking just the ingredients you need.

As we shall see in chapters 5 and 6, echinacea also may be able to relieve some of the symptoms of colds and flus.

What About Antibiotics?

Contrary to popular belief, antibiotics are not useful for colds and flus. Antibiotics kill bacteria, not viruses. In the past, people often died of bacterial infections such as bacterial pneumonia and plague, which we now easily treat with antibiotics. However, antibiotics are completely ineffective against colds and flu that are caused by viruses. Interestingly, zinc lozenges may be able to kill or at least inhibit cold viruses in the throat (see chapter 9 for more details).

Despite the fact that antibiotics do not kill viruses, people often go to the doctor and demand antibiotics—and sometimes get them—for the treatment of common viral infections. These patients may even claim that the antibiotics help (although what they are experiencing is probably the placebo effect). This misuse of antibiotics has contributed to the development of "superbugs," bacteria that are resistant to many or even all antibiotics.

Antibiotics are not useful for colds and flus.

The only situation where antibiotics are appropriate for colds is that in which a person initially infected with a viral infection *also* contracts a bacterial infection. Medical authorities strongly recommend (and even beg!) doctors and patients to limit antibiotic use to cases in which antibiotics are truly necessary.

Sometimes doctors assume that patients will insist on antibiotics, so they prescribe them as a matter of course. By telling your doctor that you want antibiotics only when absolutely necessary, you'll be doing your part to keep these vital drugs effective when they are really needed.

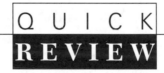

QUICK REVIEW

- Conventional medicine has much to offer, especially in the prevention and early treatment of the flu. The common cold, however, has proven difficult to prevent or treat.

- Flu vaccinations help many people avoid getting the flu in the first place and thus can be especially helpful to those at high risk for serious complications.

- When taken early enough, the medications rimantadine and amantadine can prevent the development of influenza A or minimize its symptoms.
- If you miss these opportunities to avoid the flu and do get sick, there are many over-the-counter medications that can relieve some of your symptoms. Analgesics (such as ibuprofen and acetaminophen), decongestants, expectorants, and cough suppressants may be the most helpful. Antihistamines offer little benefit.
- Antibiotics kill bacteria but are *not* appropriate for virus-caused colds and flus. They may become beneficial should you develop complications that include bacterial infections.

Echinacea and Colds and Flus

The Scientific Evidence

Remember the old saying, a cold lasts 7 days, but if you take care of yourself, you can get over it in a week? Well, it looks like with echinacea, you can actually do better. In this chapter, we'll discuss the scientific evidence that echinacea can help you get over a cold significantly faster. The herb can also make the symptoms of your cold milder and, as a bonus, may even give you some chance of not developing a full-blown cold at all. However, contrary to what you may have read, daily use of echinacea throughout the winter probably won't stop you from getting sick.

In the previous chapter, we explained some of the conventional treatments for colds and flus. In this chapter, we'll look at the research that supports taking echinacea when you get a cold or mild flu. Doctors in Europe and here in the United States and Canada have used echinacea for years to treat colds and mild flus, as well as a few other conditions.

There has been a great deal of research into this promising herb. Although echinacea is not yet a solidly proven treatment like some other herbal remedies discussed in THE NATURAL PHARMACIST series, the amount of research on it is constantly growing. Before we explain the echinacea studies, we need to explain the basics of research in general. Once you understand this information, you'll be able to evaluate any medical research you read about in books or in the news, and you'll understand the rest of this chapter better.

What Is a Double-Blind Study?

Determining whether a treatment really works is not as easy as you might think. The biggest problem is the confusing influence of the power of suggestion. If I were to give you a sugar pill and tell you it would make you feel better, chances are good that you would feel better. This so-called placebo effect is surprisingly powerful. For some conditions, such as menopausal symptoms or prostate disease, placebo treatment can essentially make symptoms disappear in as many as 50% of people.[1] While nothing is wrong with healing diseases with placebos (in fact, a lot is right with the method), this phenomenon makes it tricky to determine how well a treatment works in itself.

The amount of research on echinacea is constantly growing.

To get around this problem, researchers use the so-called *blinded placebo-controlled study*. Half the patients involved in the study are given real treatment (the treatment group), while the other half are given phony treatment (the placebo control group), and all patients are kept in the dark (they are "blind") about which group they are in. This technique factors out the power of suggestion. If the treatment group does better than the placebo control group, then researchers can conclude that the treatment really works.

It's also important to make sure that the doctor dispensing the pills doesn't know who is in which group. Doctors who are confident that they are giving a real treatment might unintentionally communicate this confidence to patients; this acts as the power of positive suggestion. They also tend to rate the results over-optimistically for the group they know is getting a medication. When both the doctor and the participant are in the dark, the experiment is considered a "double-blind" experiment. This way, the element of suggestion is eliminated. Generally speaking, we can trust only double-blind trials; we must consider the results of other types of studies contaminated by the mysterious power of the placebo effect.

Keeping the subjects "blind" is very important, but it can be tricky. For example, the smell and taste of a liquid preparation of echinacea (and some other herbs) is distinctive. Creating a substance that looks and tastes similar but has no active ingredients is difficult. This means that it's possible for those in the treatment group to know they are taking the real thing and for those in the control group to know they are taking placebo. Similar problems occur in studies of conventional medications. If a treatment causes side effects, participants and physicians may be able to tell whether they are part of the verum (treated) group rather than the placebo (untreated) group. A reliable study will report on efforts to keep the subjects "blind."

Statistics Matter

We've said that only double-blind trials are reliable. However, there is one further requirement: *statistical*

Interpreting a Study

A widely quoted study involved 50,000 people given ginseng at a Soviet auto plant. The researchers reported that participants stayed much healthier than in previous years when they were not given ginseng. Does this study mean anything?

Despite the enormous number of people who were enrolled in this study, the outcome says nothing at all.

First, no employees were *not* given ginseng (there was no control group). What if the winter when the test was given was much milder than average? Participants might have stayed healthier for *that* reason, not because they were given ginseng. A control group would have shown whether the ginseng itself, rather than some other condition, was making a difference.

---

significance. This is a very important concept to understand when you read studies.

Sometimes you will read that people in the treatment group did better than those in the placebo group, but that the results were not statistically significant. This means you cannot assume that the results proved the treatment was effective. Statistical significance is a mathematical technique used to ensure that the apparent improvement seen in the treated group represents a genuine difference, rather than just chance.

Consider the following analogy: Suppose you flip one coin 20 times and end up with 9 heads. Then, you flip a second coin 20 times and count 12 heads. Does this mean that the first coin is less likely to fall with the head side up than the second coin? Or was the difference just due to chance? A special mathematical technique can help an-

Second, the study wasn't blinded. The participants knew they were receiving ginseng. This knowledge in itself, via the power of suggestion, could have been enough to make them remain healthier. The mind is a powerful force for health.

Furthermore, the researchers knew that the participants were being treated. They would naturally be inclined to report positive results.

Only a double-blind study can tell us whether ginseng, or any other treatment, is truly effective. Fortunately, researchers have performed some double-blind studies of echinacea.

swer this question. Similarly, if a group of 20 patients take echinacea, and 9 of them catch cold, while another group of 20 take placebo and 12 of them catch cold, a mathematical technique can tell us whether this represents a true difference or is just the effect of chance. The bottom line is that when study results look good but aren't statistically significant, they can't be taken any more seriously than the apparent "bias" of the coin that happens to fall heads more often when you flip it a few times.

In Vivo Versus *In Vitro*

The factors we've just discussed are not all you must consider in evaluating the relevance of a study. Studies that use living creatures—people or animals—are called *in vivo* studies. Human studies are most meaningful to humans. Although studies in animals can give us a lot of information, animals are different from people; therefore, the results don't always transfer.

Other studies, called *in vitro* studies, are performed in test tubes. Researchers may take human cells, grow large populations of them, and then expose them to medicines, toxic substances, or anything else to be studied. Even when these tests use human cells, they do not study those cells as they function in the whole context of the human body; therefore, their results have to be taken as highly preliminary as far as how the substances tested might behave in the human body.

Most echinacea studies come from Germany, where the herb is a commonly prescribed medicine.

The reason we have discussed the nature of studies at length is that much of the research information on echinacea, while interesting, can't be taken as scientific proof that the herb is an effective treatment, simply because of the quality of the studies. Nonetheless, these studies are widely quoted, as if they actually prove something. Understanding these details of research methods will help you understand why the studies aren't as helpful as they could be. We will begin our discussion of the research on echinacea with the best studies, the double-blind placebo-controlled studies, for these are the most relevant for our purposes.

Echinacea: The Clinical Studies

Many clinical studies have focused on echinacea. Most of these come from Germany, where echinacea is a commonly prescribed medicine.

By 1994, at least 26 controlled clinical studies of the effects of echinacea had been completed, 11 of which were double blind.[2] Most of these studies examined echinacea with respect to "upper respiratory tract infections," which means illnesses involving the nose, throat, and bronchi. Colds and flus are upper respiratory tract infections. All together, these studies make a relatively good case that echinacea can reduce the number of days of sickness and make the cold and flu symptoms milder. However, the evidence that echinacea can actually *prevent* colds is weak.

Treatment of Colds and Flus

In one study, 100 people with acute upper respiratory tract infections (URIs) were divided into two groups. The members of one group took a combination product that was mostly *E. angustifolia* for 6 days, while those in the other group took placebo. All participants were examined on admission to the study, again at 2 to 4 days, and again 6 to 8 days after the start of their medication. Participants were asked to report on symptoms such as fatigue, limb pain, headache, runny nose, cough, and sore throat. While both groups improved by day 8 (as would be expected with any uncomplicated cold or flu), the echinacea group reported a decrease in all symptoms, while only some symptoms had improved in the placebo group. This difference was statistically significant for the symptoms of sore throat, runny nose, and cough, which means that the improvement was very likely due to their taking echinacea.[3]

In one study, *Echinacea angustifolia* reduced cold symptoms.

Thus though echinacea did not cure the common cold, the herb did decrease cold symptoms. Unfortunately, this study involved *E. angustifolia* rather than *E. purpurea*. As you may recall from chapter 1, *E. purpurea* is the most commonly available variety of the herb in North America, though you can find products that contain the *angustifolia* variety, or sometimes both varieties together.

Another double-blind placebo-controlled study followed 160 adults with recent onset of an upper respiratory infection.[4] Patients were given *E. pallida* or placebo for 10 days. The results showed a statistically significant reduction in the duration of illness, from 13 days in the placebo group to about 9.5 days in the treated group. Again, this study did not use the more commonly available *E. purpurea*.

In double-blind studies of people with colds or flus, both *E. pallida* and *E. purpurea* have reduced the length of the illness.

A slightly larger double-blind placebo-controlled study followed 180 people using an alcohol extract of *E. purpurea* roots, much like preparations that are available in North America.[5] This study involved one group taking 90 drops (450 mg, or about 0.75 teaspoon) of echinacea daily, a second group taking 180 drops (900 mg, or about 1.5 teaspoon), and a third group taking placebo. The researchers' intent was to determine whether dosage could alter the efficacy of echinacea. The researchers evaluated participants at the onset of treatment, again at 3 to 4 days, and again at 8 to 10 days, looking for indications that echinacea shortened the duration or severity of colds.

This study found that the group given 90 drops of echinacea tincture daily did not show significant improvements when compared to the placebo group. However, in the group taking the larger, 180-drop dose, there was a statistically significant improvement in severity and duration of cold symptoms.

Finding better results with a higher dose of a treatment (technically called a "dose-related response") is a good sign. It is generally a strong indication that a treatment is actually effective.

Prevention of Colds and Flus

The studies just described tell us that echinacea may help reduce the symptoms of colds; they don't, however, tell us whether echinacea can prevent colds.

Another study suggested that echinacea can sometimes stop a cold that is just starting. In this study, 120 people were given *E. purpurea* or placebo as soon as they started showing signs of getting a cold. This study was double blinded and lasted for a total of 10 days after each person started taking either the echinacea or the placebo.[6]

A double-blind study found that *E. purpurea* can sometimes stop a cold that is just starting.

Participants took either echinacea or the placebo at a dose of 20 drops every 2 hours for 1 day, then 20 drops 3 times per day for 9 more days. The results were promising. First, fewer people in the echinacea group felt that their initial symptoms actually developed into "real" colds (40% of those taking echinacea versus 60% taking the placebo actually became ill). Second, among those who did come down with "real" colds, improvement in the symptoms started sooner in the echinacea group (starting at 4 days instead

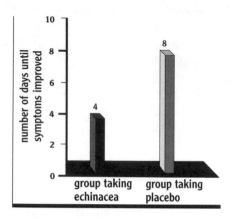

Figure 3. *Double-blind study shows that echinacea can help you feel better faster* (Hoheisel et al., 1997)

of 8 days—see figure 3). Both of these results were statistically significant.

A different double-blind placebo-controlled study attempted to discover whether echinacea can prevent infections from even starting.[7] This 8-week study included 108 people, 54 of whom took *E. purpurea* and 54 of whom did not. This study examined not only cold symptoms but also specific immune system effects that can be studied objectively—for example, the total number of white blood cells and the ratio of different white cells (T4 and T8 cells). All participants admitted to the study were considered at increased risk for infections, based on criteria such as their having had at least three upper respiratory tract infections or URI-related complications during the previous winter.

The results from this study were promising but not definitive. Echinacea did not entirely prevent colds; some people taking echinacea did get sick. The treated group did get fewer colds, but the difference when compared to the control group was not statistically significant. Those in the treated group also experienced a longer period of health before the first cold—40 versus 25 days. Unfortunately, while this study is widely misquoted as clear evidence that echinacea is effective, from a mathematical point of view, these findings cannot be considered significant. This study simply doesn't tell us much.

For those who get sick especially easily, the regular use of echinacea may slightly decrease the number of winter colds.

Similar results were found in a more recent and larger study.[8] In this double-blind placebo-controlled trial, 302 healthy volunteers were given an alcohol tincture containing either *E. purpurea* root, *E. angustifolia* root, or placebo for a period of 12 weeks. The results showed that *E. purpurea* was associated with perhaps a 20% decrease in the number of people who got sick, and *E. angustifolia* with a 10% decrease. However, once again, the difference was not statistically significant. The problem is that the benefit, if any, was so small that it could have been due to chance alone.

Statistically significant benefits were seen in another double-blind placebo-controlled study, at least for those especially likely to catch cold.[9] The study involved 609 students at the University of Cologne. Half the participants were treated with a German product containing *E. angustifolia* for at least 8 weeks; the other half received placebo.

Why Good Studies of Herbal Medicines Are Difficult to Come By

Drugs are regulated by the Food and Drug Administration (FDA). This governmental body makes every effort to ensure that the drugs we use are safe, effective, and used appropriately. Pharmaceutical companies are required to perform many tests on their new drugs long before they can put them on the market. All together, these tests are extremely expensive, taking 5 to 12 years and costing hundreds of millions of dollars for each new drug. The only reason drug manufacturers can afford to spend this kind of money is that they expect to make it back by owning the patent on the drug.

Herbs are in a different situation. It is possible to skip some research steps with them, because they are already in wide

In the group as a whole, echinacea did not significantly decrease the number of colds. However, of the total group studied, 363 students were rated as particularly infection-prone, based on the number of infections each had developed the winter before. This relatively high-risk group *did* show a statistically significant reduction in the total number of colds when compared with the control group. The change, while not gigantic, was significant: The infection-prone students developed on average 20% fewer colds. This study does indicate that, for those who get sick especially easily, the regular use of echinacea may slightly decrease the number of winter colds. However, the bottom line is that echinacea is not very effective (if at all) as a long-term preventive treatment. It is better used right at the onset of a cold to reduce its severity and duration or, with luck, to ward it off entirely.

use, and you don't have to start with animals to prove that they are safe to take. However, herbs cannot be patented. When one supplement manufacturer pays to research an herbal remedy, every other manufacturer uses that research to sell their own herbal supplements. The manufacturer who paid for the costly research does not gain a unique advantage from the research dollars spent. This has restricted research into herbal medicine as well as other natural supplements.

In Germany herbal manufacturers have funded such studies anyway, and they use the results to increase product sales. American herbal companies are beginning to follow suit.

Echinacea: Laboratory Studies

The double-blind studies just described strongly indicate that echinacea can reduce the severity and duration of colds and suggest that it can help prevent colds as well. Other studies have examined echinacea's ability to affect a variety of immune system measures of activity in test tubes or in the human body. These laboratory studies are interesting, and many show that echinacea can stimulate the immune system. However, they are not directly clinically applicable, and we don't yet know whether they imply a meaningful change in immunity. For this reason, our discussion of them will be brief.

One study showed that both injected and oral administration of echinacea caused an increase in phagocytosis.[10] As you may recall from chapter 2, *phagocytosis* is the swallowing of foreign bodies by white blood cells. In this study, phagocytosis increased while echinacea was administered and returned to normal within a few days after echinacea was stopped.

This is an interesting result. It may indicate that echinacea somehow arouses white blood cells and puts them on the alert, perhaps because some component of echinacea resembles a dangerous foreign body. Or this phenomenon could indicate that echinacea stimulates white blood cells. We'll discuss these hypotheses more in the next chapter.

Animal and test tube studies have also found evidence that echinacea increases white blood cell activity.[11–17] Unfortunately, an increase in measured levels of phagocytosis may or may not translate into any meaningful effect on immunity as a whole. A good analogy might be when a certain football coach gets his players to run faster and jump up and down more vigorously in practice. This may be a good sign, but the proof of his effectiveness doesn't come until the team wins more games.

The bottom line: Echinacea is not very effective (if at all) as a long-term preventive treatment. It is better used right at the onset of a cold to lessen symptoms and reduce the number of days you're sick.

In this case, the bottom line is fewer infections. To determine whether or not taking echinacea produces this result, we need more clinical studies like those described above.

How Does Echinacea Work?

The simplest answer to the question of how echinacea works is "We don't know."

Human research evidence suggests that echinacea increases what is called *cell-mediated immunity*. This is the part of the immune system involving T-lymphocytes. Doctors can test this type of immunity using an injection under the skin. For instance, the tuberculosis test called PPD checks to see whether you have cell-mediated immunity against the TB bacillus. If you do, it means that you've been exposed and might need treatment. Sometimes, doctors give a similar skin test checking for cell-mediated immunity against common infections such as measles. In this case the assumption is that you've been exposed (to either the real disease or a vaccine), so you should show a reaction to this test. If you don't react, it may be that your immune system is simply "sleepy." (The scientific name for this immune laziness is "anergy.")

In one study, echinacea extracts were found to "wake up" the immune system and increase the reaction in tests of cell-mediated immunity.[18] This strongly suggests that echinacea is an immune stimulant.

However, we don't know what component in echinacea is responsible. Polysaccharides have gotten a lot of attention as possible active constituents of echinacea. Some theorists have

In one study, echinacea extracts were found to "wake up" the immune system.

hypothesized that echinacea's polysaccharides resemble compounds similar to those found in bacteria. The human immune system, confronted with these substances, may believe itself under attack and build up its defensive activity. There are many polysaccharides found in echinacea. These polysaccharides have been shown to stimulate t-lymphocytes and macrophages. In particular, they increase macrophage anti-tumor activity *in vitro*. It has also been shown that some polysaccharides can increase the ability of macrophages to produce chemicals that can stimulate increased activity from other cells in the immune system.[19,20,21]

The problem with this theory is that echinacea polysaccharides do not seem to be present in significant concentrations in echinacea products, and some question exists about their ability to survive in the intestines long enough to be absorbed.[22]

Cichoric acid is another promising candidate. It is actually found in both alcoholic extracts of echinacea and the dried herb. It exists in preparations made from the fresh plant as well, but in varying degrees. This is because certain enzymes in the fresh plant can degrade cichoric acid over time.[23] Cichoric acid has been found in test tube and animal experiments to increase white blood cell activity.

Echinacea's fat-soluble components, polyacetylenes and alkylamides, most common in the roots, have also exhibited immune-stimulating activity in animal and test tube studies[24] and may be among the most active of echinacea's ingredients.[25]

A final point: Many people who talk about echinacea say that it strengthens the immune system. Unfortunately, no scientific evidence supports this theory. It is at least as likely that echinacea simply stimulates the immune system into increased action, perhaps by simulating the response to components of actual antigens. Such stimulation is a far cry from "strengthening" and might not always be good for you since an excessively active immune system can cause numerous health problems. This is the reason echinacea is not recommended in autoimmune diseases (see chapter 7 for more information).

Not Just for Colds and Flus

Most clinical use of echinacea focuses on colds and flus, but this herb has been used for other illnesses too.

For example, studies have examined echinacea's ability to fight the common yeast *Candida albicans.* This yeast can infect the GI tract (causing thrush) and the vagina (causing vaginal yeast infections).

One study involved 203 women with vaginal yeast infections given various forms of echinacea for 10 weeks, along with a standard yeast infection treatment.[26] The results indicate that echinacea can improve the effectiveness of conventional anti-fungal medications. Unfortunately, because the study was not blinded, how much of the outcome was due to the power of suggestion is unclear.

Echinacea has also been studied for its wound-healing ability. Several studies have found that echinacea can decrease inflammation in animals and promote wound healing.[27–31] However, none of these studies meet current scientific standards, so they can't be viewed as proof that echinacea helps heal wounds.

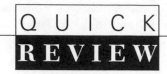

- Although the research record is not complete, evidence suggests that echinacea can reduce the number of days a cold lasts and make the symptoms more mild.

- Echinacea may also reduce the number of colds per year you get if taken at the first sign of symptoms.

- Echinacea is not very effective (if at all) as a long-term preventive treatment.

- Although we don't know how echinacea works, intriguing studies suggest that it affects aspects of the immune system. We can't say exactly what echinacea does, or if it actually stimulates the immune system.

- It is clear that echinacea has an effect on our bodies when we have infections and that it somehow helps people get better faster.

How to Use and Purchase Echinacea

I n this chapter, we'll tell you how much echinacea you should use, and how and where to purchase it. In the next chapter, we'll explain everything you need to know about the safety of using echinacea so that you can completely understand how to use it on your own.

Dosage

When you decide to take echinacea, you have a few variables to consider because it comes in different forms. The short list on the next page gives you general guidelines for dosages of the most common forms of echinacea, whether derived from *E. purpurea, E. angustifolia, E. pallida,* or some mix of the three.

However, these dosage recommendations are only approximations. While starting with the most commonly used dosage is generally best, you may find you need to take more or less, depending on your personal medical and physical situation. Echinacea's excellent safety record means you can comfortably experiment with the dose until you find what works best for you. When in doubt, consult a qualified health-care practitioner.

Dried root: 0.5 to 1 gram 3 times per day

Juice: 2 to 3 ml ($\frac{1}{2}$ to $\frac{3}{4}$ teaspoon*) 3 times per day

Tincture 1:5** : 2 to 4 ml ($\frac{1}{2}$ to 1 teaspoon) 3 times per day

Fluid extract 1:1: 1 to 2 ml ($\frac{1}{4}$ to $\frac{1}{2}$ teaspoon) 3 times per day

Dry, powdered extract (standardized to 3.5% echinacoside): 300 mg 3 times per day

Freeze-dried: 1 to 2 capsules or tablets 3 times per day

One Family's Story

Consider the experience of Anne, a patient of mine. She lives about 45 minutes from my office, and getting in with her four kids is a major endeavor. After considerable experience with her own kids and some effort to learn about the basic childhood illnesses, Anne can tell the difference between a common cold and something more serious.

When one of Anne's kids gets a cold or flu, she shifts into high gear. She begins giving echinacea to all her kids (not to mention herself and her spouse), makes sure they drink plenty of fluids, and keeps her eye out for complications. When she brings the children in for their annual school physicals, Anne picks up enough of her kids' favorite echinacea to get through the first cold or two in the fall, and she stocks up on more whenever she's in town. Does it help? Anne thinks it does, and based on the scientific evidence described in the last chapter, she's probably right.

---

*Note that $\frac{1}{2}$ teaspoon = 60 drops

**Indicates the ratio of plant to liquid, which should be clearly marked on all tinctures or extracts you purchase

How Long Should You Take Echinacea?

There is no clear-cut answer to this question, and it remains a matter of some controversy.

In a study discussed earlier, participants stopped taking echinacea when they felt better and didn't think they needed it anymore, and did not report feeling worse again.[1] This study suggests that it is okay to stop taking echinacea once you feel better. The case is very different for antibiotics, where it is generally advised that you take the antibiotics for the prescribed time, even if your symptoms disappear before you finish the medicine (which they usually do). I generally suggest that people keep taking echinacea for 1 day after they feel better again.

Echinacea's excellent safety record means you can comfortably experiment with the dose until you find what works best for you.

Most research has studied people taking echinacea for 7 to 10 days, the usual duration of an average cold or flu. Taking echinacca for this long is certainly safe and reasonable. If you are still suffering from mild symptoms after 7 days, keep taking your echinacea for a few more days, until you feel completely better. If, after 7 to 10 days, you aren't feeling considerably better, get to the doctor; you may have something more serious than just a cold.

There are some who believe that echinacea should never be taken for more than 8 weeks or that you should take "breaks," going off the medication if you are taking it for more than a couple of weeks at a time. These issues are discussed in the next chapter.

What Doctors and Herbalists Say

Most practitioners educated in herbal medicine use echinacea often and with great confidence and comfort.

In the pharmacy at my clinic in Portland, we have more than a dozen different types of products using echinacea. We carry it in virtually every form available, from capsules to liquids to salves. We stock more sizes and varieties of echinacea preparations than any other product in our pharmacy, and we use them all.

Some people may use echinacea all winter long, while others use it only when they feel a cold coming on. However, because clinical research offers little to no support for the use of echinacea as a cold prevention tool, and taking any medication when you aren't sick is questionable, we suggest using echinacea only when you feel that cold creeping up on you.

Herbal practitioners report a variety of ways they use echinacea.

Make a tea. One colleague suggested making echinacea tea and having kids over the age of 2 and susceptible adults (those who are prone to getting colds) drink one or two cups a day in hope of benefiting from echinacea before the colds take hold.

The taste can be partially masked with diluted fruit juice or with a flavored tea.

Taper the dose. Another common suggestion, and the one I use most with my patients, is to take more at the beginning of your cold, then to taper off after a couple of days. Most of my colleagues recommend taking echinacea every 2 hours for about 2 days, then taking it 3 to 4 times per day until the cold resolves. Even though they didn't all agree on what dose was best, all agreed that taking it this way was a good idea.

Take at onset of cold. Start taking echinacea at the first sign of a cold. Because there doesn't seem to be any real risk in taking echinacea for a few days if you don't need it, don't hesitate and don't wonder. If you think you might be getting sick, take echinacea for a couple of days until you know, one way or the other. If you do get sick, keep taking it; if you don't, you can stop. If you get very sick, and echinacea isn't helping you, see your doctor.

Echinacea appears to be most beneficial when taken early.

One point of agreement among all the doctors we spoke to is that people should keep echinacea on hand and know in advance how to use it. Echinacea appears to be most beneficial when taken early. Once you're definitely sick, you won't notice as much benefit from taking echinacea.

What to Expect from Echinacea

Echinacea tends to produce *gradual* results. Don't expect to wake up after having taken one dose of echinacea and be completely free of cold symptoms. If you take echinacea as you feel a cold coming on, you can expect to have a shorter and less severe cold than you usually do. Taking echinacea may reduce your horribly stuffy nose to mild congestion. If you usually progress from a stuffy chest to a bad cough, echinacea may help reduce the chest congestion so you avoid the cough. It isn't magic, but it can help.

Sarah, a mother of two children under three, complained that her colds had gotten worse since she had kids. After we talked about echinacea, she decided to try it.

When she felt her next cold coming on, she took the echinacea as we discussed (every 2 hours for the first 2 days, then less often, as described above). She still got a runny nose and sore throat but said she could keep up with her kids through the entire cold and that her symptoms were only bad for about a day. This was a big improvement for her, and she was almost eager for her next cold to see whether echinacea would help her again (not an attitude I'd necessarily recommend). When her next cold came around, she was equally diligent about taking her echinacea and reported that her cold was even milder than the previous one. Sarah was thrilled, and now she uses echinacea for everyone in her family as soon as she hears any sniffles.

Echinacea tends to produce *gradual* results.

Echinacea does not always work this well, however, and compared to the studies discussed in the last chapter, Sarah's results were better than average.

Tom didn't fare so well. Even though he followed my instructions, he found the results disappointing. He thought his head might be less stuffy, but he still had to carry tissues for his runny nose, so the improvement didn't make much difference to him. He hadn't had a fever to begin with, and his sore throat hadn't changed at all. After a couple of days on echinacea, he came in to see me. I tried some of the other approaches described in chapters 8 and 9, and he began to improve, although it could have been that his cold was getting ready to go away anyway. This herb is definitely not a cure-all; it performs better some times than others. Still, for those who get good results, echinacea is a must-have.

One Difference Between Herbs and Drugs

Buying herbal products need not be difficult or confusing, although it is not as easy as buying drugs. Whether you buy extra-strength Tylenol or a generic brand of extra-strength acetaminophen, you're getting 500 mg of acetaminophen per pill. This sort of consistency makes buying products like acetaminophen easy. Echinacea, as you may have already discovered, comes in a lot of different types of products and strengths, and we do not know which ones are best.

While this uncertainty is irritating, it isn't necessarily dangerous. Echinacea is a safe enough product that you can feel free to experiment until you find what works best for you. *Warning:* With herbs, as elsewhere, quality matters. Many people simply buy the cheapest product available, but this is not necessarily a good idea. The Food and Drug Administration regulates herbal medicines as dietary supplements, not as medicines, which means that there is very little oversight of product quality. You need to do some of the footwork and make sure you are using a reputable brand. The best source of information is a qualified health-care practitioner.

Finally, once you find a brand that you like—one that works for you—stick with it. By shopping for a bargain, you may get an inferior product and end up wasting your money and not helping your cold.

Does Form Dictate Function?

Now you're ready to buy your echinacea, right? Not quite. When you go to buy your echinacea, you'll find yourself confronted by many possible forms of echinacea, including tinctures, tablets, capsules, salves, teas and creams.

Be a Careful Consumer

Many people who take herbal medicines are concerned about what they eat and drink. Often, people want to avoid pesticides or animal products, which can be difficult if you aren't familiar with a manufacturer's products.

If you are concerned about any ingredients, either because you are allergic to something like corn or because you are a vegetarian and prefer not to take gelatin capsules, you can take a few precautions to make sure you don't get ingredients you don't want.

- **Read the label.** Carefully. There is often a statement of what *isn't* in a product. For example, "Contains no sugar, yeast, corn, wheat, or dairy products" is a common statement.

How do you choose the right one for you? While there is no "right" when it comes to your choosing what to take, the task is simpler than it may appear. Once you know what type of product you like, stick with it, and all your future purchases will be easy.

Tablets and capsules are the most convenient for most people. However, some people and many professionals prefer tinctures. One advantage is that you can easily combine several tinctures into a formula; this flexibility is why naturopaths and other herbalists like them. If you like using echinacea and would like to try other herbs (such as those mentioned in chapter 8), you might buy tinctures and try combining them to see whether you get better results. (*Note:* The safety or efficacy of herbal combinations has, for the most part, not been evaluated.)

- **Learn about by-products.** This is just like reading food labels. If something says high-fructose syrup, that probably means corn. Vegetable starch is commonly made from corn or potatoes. If it doesn't say "vegetarian," those capsules may not be from a vegetable source, but rather gelatin.
- **Call the manufacturer.** When in any doubt, go to the only source that can always tell you what you need to know. I once had a concerned patient who wanted to avoid corn, so I called the manufacturer to find out which vegetable they used to get the vegetable glycerine in their herbal glycerites. The manufacturer should be able and willing to answer your questions. If the company that made a particular product isn't, buy from someone else.

People frequently object to the taste of tinctures, and some do not want the alcohol. To avoid the taste of tinctures, you can get empty capsules (at pharmacies and health-food stores), put your tinctures into them, then swallow them fast— before the capsules dissolve. If it's the alcohol you dislike, and you can't find another form of echinacea, you can evaporate the alcohol. Simply put the tincture into a glass and add between $\frac{1}{8}$ and $\frac{1}{4}$ cup of boiling water. When it's cooled, the alcohol will be mostly gone.

When you find a form and brand of echinacea you like and that works for you, stick with it.

What's in a Package?

You'll feel a lot more comfortable choosing an herbal medicine if you have an idea of what you'll find when you get to the store, not to mention an idea of what you want. To assist you in making your choice, here's a basic glossary of the most common forms of herbal medicines. Keep in mind that you may need to try several types before you find your favorites.

capsule. Dry herb, with or without other ingredients, crushed and put into a gelatin or vegetable capsule. Dry extracts can also be placed in capsules.

fluid extract. An extract of a plant using one part liquid (often alcohol or water) to one part plant material. These are stronger than tincture, and usually have a consistency similar to that of honey.

Another trick I frequently use is masking the flavor with grape juice. Purple grape juice masks almost any flavor, so I recommend adding a small amount to a dose of a tincture to make it palatable. Some of my patients keep frozen grape juice concentrate in the freezer for just such occasions, spooning out a tiny bit (about a $1/4$ teaspoon) when they need it.

Some herbalists prefer liquids, saying that swallowing the tincture allows the echinacea to bathe the lymph glands in the throat. This, they believe, helps trigger the immune system. However, if you can't stand the liquids, you can always buy echinacea in capsules or tablets.

You can also find combinations of herbs (like echinacea with ginger) and vitamins (maybe vitamins A and C

glycerite. An extract made using glycerine as the solvent rather than alcohol or water. The final product is thicker than a tincture, about the consistency of syrup. Glycerites are sweet and often used for children.

tablet. Herbs or dry extracts, perhaps with other ingredients like vitamins and minerals, pressed together into a tablet. Tableting agents, usually inert ingredients, are used to make the blend hold a shape.

tincture. An herbal extract made using alcohol or alcohol and water to extract chemicals from raw or dry herbs. Strengths vary from 1:5 to 1:10 (plant:liquid). Alcohol content varies, too.

with echinacea) in capsules and tablets. These can be convenient if you know how to use them, but do be careful if you are not familiar with the formula. Read the label carefully and talk to a physician or pharmacist trained in herbal remedies to be sure you aren't getting ingredients you don't need. For example, some of the vitamins included can become toxic at large doses. If you take echinacea every 2 hours at the beginning of a cold, you might exceed the safe range of an included vitamin. A different problem is that you may be wasting your money on unnecessary ingredients. For example, although echinacea is often sold in combination with the expensive herb goldenseal, there is no evidence that goldenseal offers any benefits when taken at the onset of a cold (see chapter 8).

Choose Your Weapon: *E. Angustifolia, E. Purpurea,* or *E. Pallida*

Choosing a species and part of echinacea can be difficult. Historically, herbalists have used the various parts and species for different types of treatments, but few of these uses have been studied scientifically. It is possible (even likely) that the various varieties work on the same symptoms, but without research that compares them, we just don't know. Is the situation similar to the cold medicine that takes care of cough and sore throat versus the one that helps with stuffy nose and headache? Probably not, but without further research, we cannot know for sure.

The clinical studies we looked at in chapter 5 are divided pretty equally between *E. purpurea* and *E. angustifolia.* It appears that all three species of echinacea—*purpurea,*[2] *angustifolia,*[3] and *pallida*[4]—can help reduce cold and flu symptoms. This should be encouraging, since not all manufacturers use the same species. Some studies have shown that alcohol extracts may be more active than water extracts, but we don't know much about dry herbs or other types of products.[5]

Ultimately, the best answer depends on your results. If you love an *E. purpurea* product but tried an *E. angustifolia* formula that didn't work for you, keep buying the *purpurea.* You'll feel more confident about it, and you'll probably have better results. Even though your choice may not be the only product that could work for you, there's no harm in playing favorites when using echinacea.

Where Do You Get It and How Much Does It Cost?

Echinacea is widely available in pharmacies, health-food stores, and many natural food stores. Depending on the form you choose, it should range from $10 to $15 per cold or flu. Liquids run about $8 to $10 per ounce, and echinacea alone in capsules is usually $8 to $10 per bottle. Some of the fancier products (containing several herbs or herbs with vitamins and minerals) may be as much as $25 per bottle.

When Not to Use Echinacea

Echinacea is not meant to be a substitute for antibiotics or other medications for serious illnesses. Even for ordinary colds and flus, if you take echinacea for more than a week and are not seeing improvement (or especially if you're getting worse), you probably don't have just a cold. In such a situation, see your doctor for a more appropriate treatment. Echinacea may also not be as effective as prescription medications for influenza A, so if you are in a high-risk group, as described in chapter 3, it might be prudent to use the medication.

Echinacea appears to be a safe herb for most people. However, there are a few safety issues that will be discussed in the next chapter.

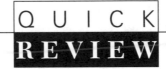

- Because there are many forms of echinacea, there isn't one specific dose that can be recommended. Typical doses for various forms are as follows:

Dried root: 0.5 to 1 g 3 times per day

Juice: 2 to 3 ml ($^1/_2$ to $^3/_4$ teaspoon) 3 times per day

Tincture (1:5): 2 to 4 ml ($^1/_2$ to 1 teaspoon) 3 times per day

Fluid extract (1:1): 1 to 2 ml ($^1/_4$ to $^1/_2$ teaspoon) 3 times per day

Dry, powdered extract (standardized to 3.5% echinacoside): 300 mg 3 times per day

Freeze-dried: 1 to 2 capsules or tablets 3 times per day

However, these dosage recommendations are only approximations. While starting with the most commonly used dosage is generally best, you may find you need to take more or less, depending on your personal medical and physical situation. Echinacea's excellent safety record means you can comfortably experiment with the dose until you find what works best for you. When in doubt, consult a qualified healthcare practitioner.

■ Most physicians who use herbal medicines recommend you start taking echinacea at the first sign of a cold and continue taking it until you feel completely better. Commonly, naturopathic physicians suggest taking 60 drops or 2 capsules/tablets every 2 hours for a day or two, then taking it 3 or 4 times per day until your cold is gone.

■ Echinacea is not a single-dose wonder cure for colds and flus. You need to take it early and take it frequently to realize any benefit from it. If you follow recommended doses, though, you may be pleased when your cold and flu symptoms are milder and don't last as long.

- When echinacea doesn't work, especially if you've been taking it for a week without results, see a physician for a full evaluation and a more appropriate treatment. Do not try to use echinacea for more serious infections.

Safety Issues

While drugs are tested for their safety and efficacy, herbal medicines do not undergo the same type of extensive formal testing because they are legally considered foods. This means we may not know as much as we would like about the safety and efficacy of herbs. However, millions of people worldwide use echinacea for their colds and flus, and few side effects have been reported. The cumulative scientific evidence from both human and animal studies also suggests that this is a very safe herb.

The Difference Between Side Effects and Toxicity

Most people have suffered side effects—unpleasant, unintended consequences—when using a medication. Some occur only rarely; others regularly accompany the use of certain products. Over-the-counter antihistamines frequently cause fatigue and mental cloudiness, and decongestants commonly cause insomnia. Certain antibiotics lead to yeast infections so reliably that doctors often prescribe anti-yeast treatment right from the start.

The cumulative scientific evidence from both human and animal studies suggests that echinacea is a very safe herb.

Side effects are general problems that can occur with almost any substance, even foods. Dairy products may produce mucus congestion, and beans and legumes almost always cause bloating and gas. It is no surprise, therefore, that herbs can cause side effects as well.

Side effects generally go away when you stop using whatever caused them, and they may occur at normal or even low doses of a treatment. We usually use a different word, *toxicity*, to refer to more serious adverse effects including actual injury to the body. Most commonly, toxic reactions occur when a substance is taken in excessive doses.

To understand the difference, compare Prozac and acetaminophen. At normal dosages, Prozac can cause insomnia, headache, nausea, sexual problems, and other unpleasant side effects. If you were to take twenty Prozac pills, however, it is likely that nothing serious would happen to you. In other words, Prozac causes numerous side effects but is not very toxic.[1]

Acetaminophen, on the other hand, seldom causes any side effects when taken at the proper dosage. If you take too much acetaminophen, though, you are likely to suffer severe or even fatal liver damage. Thus acetaminophen causes few side effects but is potentially toxic.

The good news about echinacea is that people who have taken it over the years report very few incidences of either side effects or toxicity.

Echinacea's Excellent Side-Effect Profile

A paper published in 1996 reviewed 2,000 patient observations from all the published studies on echinacea.[2] The reviewer found no serious side effects among the participants, some of whom took echinacea for up to 12 weeks. Minor side effects that were reported included the following.

Oral effects. The most common "adverse reaction" (reported by 5% of those studied) was an unpleasant taste.[3] Some also noted a warm or tingling feeling in their mouth when they first took echinacea. This sensation, caused by the alkylamides in the *purpurea*

> **Few side effects have been reported by people using echinacea.**

and *angustifolia* varieties, usually dissipates quickly after you take a dose but will return with each successive dose.[4]

Digestive upset. Burping, bloating, and flatulence have been associated with large doses of echinacea. In one study some users (0.24%) noted a laxative effect within the first 48 hours of taking large doses (500 to 1,000 mg of *angustifolia*); this does stop after the first 48 hours. Some people (0.48%) reported nausea, and a few (0.24%) noted abdominal pain.[5]

Urinary tract effects. Echinacea sometimes produces a slight increase in urination, which disappears after the first 2 days.[6]

Allergic reactions. One article from Australia noted that a woman with a strong personal history of allergies had an anaphylactic reaction to echinacea.[7] (An anaphylactic reaction is what a person experiences who has a severe life-threatening allergy to something such as bee stings, shrimp, or strawberries. An anaphylactic reaction is basically an exaggeration of a normal allergic response and can lead to death in under an hour. An epinephrine injection usually reverses the process almost immediately.) The woman's doctor did a standard skin-prick allergy test and found that she was hypersensitive to echinacea. While this sort of reaction can occur with any herb or drug, such reactions appear to be relatively rare with echinacea.

Out of thousands of patients, I have seen only two patients who had allergic reactions to herbs. Although echinacea was not the trigger in either case, both herbs that did cause these reactions have a similar reputation for being very safe. I have also used both of the products that caused the reactions with patients many times before and since, without any adverse effects. It shows you the unpredictable nature of allergies.

Consider the story of Carla, who had come in for a general checkup. When routine blood tests indicated that she was mildly anemic, I prescribed an herbal combination for anemia that I had used many times, supplied by a manufacturer I trust. She called me the next morning, not sure whether she was reacting to the herbs or to something else. She felt okay, but her lips were swollen. I asked whether she had been exposed to anything new, other than the herbs, and whether she had any known allergies. When she answered no in both cases, I told her to stop taking the herbs and to take an over-the-counter antihistamine. The swelling (a condition called angioedema) disappeared and never returned. Carla, of course, didn't take any more of that particular product.

Angioedema is basically a variety of hives. It can be dangerous if it involves the tongue and throat or escalates into an anaphylactic reaction.

If you have a severe allergic reaction to an herb, don't take it again. As with bee sting and other severe allergies, each successive reaction is usually worse than the one before. However, although the symptoms of such allergies are dramatic, they don't mean that the herb (or drug) that caused them is a dangerous treatment, any more than shrimp or strawberries are dangerous foods.

Toxicity

Echinacea seems to be a very nontoxic substance. Despite the widespread use of echinacea in Europe, no serious adverse effects have been reported. According to one highly respected German text: "The oral use of echinacea is considered to be without significant toxicologic risk."[8]

To fully determine the safety of a substance, researchers typically go through a formal process: they give the substance to animals, including pregnant animals, for months or even years at various doses and look for adverse effects. They check to see if it causes death or significant

Echinacea seems to be a very non-toxic substance.

diseases such as cancer, or if it produces birth defects. When evaluating herbs, researchers also study the effects of each individual chemical, separate from the plant as a whole.

This formal process has not yet been completed for echinacea. However, what research has been performed supports the impression that this is a safe herb. In one study, researchers gave both rats and mice *E. purpurea* at doses that correspond to "many times the human therapeutic dose," and results showed no evidence of toxicity.[9] Other studies have found that echinacea did not cause mutations or demonstrate cancer-causing properties.

Studies focusing on echinacea's polysaccharides (large sugar molecules that may contribute to its immune stimu-

Conditions That Warrant Special Caution

Echinacea's status as a possible immune system stimulant makes its use potentially risky for those with certain medical conditions. In general these are conditions in which, for some reason, the immune system (all or part of it) is already overactive and might not respond to echinacea in a beneficial way. Such conditions include:

- AIDS
- Leukemia
- Auto-immune diseases
- Tuberculosis
- Rheumatoid arthritis

lation) have also found them to be nontoxic. Echinacea does contain substances known as pyrrolizidine alkaloids that can be toxic to the liver, but the particular type found in echinacea is not dangerous.[10]

Theoretical Warnings

A special governmental committee in Germany (Commission E) recommends caution when using echinacea if you have certain medical conditions. These cautions are based on theoretical concerns. It isn't that any actual harm due to echinacea use has been observed in people with these conditions (listed below). Rather, there are reasons to believe harm might be possible.

Autoimmune Diseases

With an autoimmune disease, the body's immune system attacks part of the body. The theoretical concern is that

- Systemic lupus erythematosus
- Hashimoto's thyroiditis
- Scleroderma
- Myasthenia gravis
- Mixed connective tissue disease
- Goodpasture's syndrome
- Pemphigus
- Sjogren's syndrome

However, no direct evidence suggests that echinacea causes harm in these conditions.

echinacea might further stimulate an already overactive immune system. While this theory is interesting, no current clinical or scientific evidence suggests that this actually occurs, and no published studies report any harm to people with autoimmune disease who took echinacea.[11] Nonetheless, autoimmune diseases are so serious that medical professionals recommend against using echinacea in these conditions.

Leukemia

Leukemia is a cancer of the bone marrow, characterized by an extremely elevated white blood cell count. Because the high white blood cell count in leukemia is part of its nature as a cancer, rather than due to an overactive immune system, it's difficult to conceive just how echinacea could affect this condition. Furthermore, one study showed no adverse effects from long-term use of echinacea by people with chronic lymphocytic leukemia, and no studies have revealed any problems associated with using echinacea in leukemia patients.[12] Nevertheless, as with autoimmune diseases, the serious nature of leukemia warrants extreme caution.

AIDS

The debate continues among herbalists about whether to use echinacea for individuals who have AIDS or are HIV-positive. Herbalist Paul Bergner somewhat sheepishly says he caused some of the doubt by suggesting that echinacea might not be appropriate for people with AIDS. He now feels that his own suggestion was erroneous. Bergner, exercising caution, based his original doubts on a 1986 study that showed a decline in the T4:T8 cell ratio in patients given echinacea injections daily for 7 days. Since the T4:T8 cell ratio is an important measure of AIDS progression, anything that lowers it would certainly be contraindicated.

Further examination of the research record convinced Bergner that this caution is valid for injected echinacea only, not for the oral echinacea used in North America. He now says that, considering the evidence of echinacea's improvements in cell-mediated immunity in those with depressed immunity, there is no reason for people with AIDS to avoid oral echinacea.[13] Nonetheless, there remain lingering concerns.

Note: Echinacea has not been found safe or helpful in treating AIDS.

Tuberculosis

Another condition in which the German Commission E recommends caution is tuberculosis. In tuberculosis, macrophages (the foreigner-gobbling patrol cells of the immune system) in the lungs try to kill the bacteria and stimulate the rest of the immune system to act against the infection. Sometimes, however, the bacteria are strong enough to live and reproduce inside the macrophages. In these cases, t-cells can recognize these infected macrophages and kill them, thus killing the tuberculosis bacteria inside them as well. However, the t-cells also break down infected lung tissue, causing considerable lung damage in the process. In some ways this accidental damage can be worse than what is caused by the TB bacillus itself.

The concern is that t-cells, if overstimulated by echinacea, might cause increased damage to the lungs. Although no experimental evidence supports this concern, anyone with tuberculosis should consult a physician before using echinacea or indeed any herb or supplement.

Long-Term Effects of Echinacea

Germany's Commission E suggests that users not take echinacea for more than 8 weeks, but it does not give a reason for this warning. It appears to be based on fears that long-term use of echinacea may suppress the immune system.

This idea seems to come from evidence that patients given high-dose echinacea injections suffer a decline in immune system response.[14] However, no evidence suggests that oral echinacea causes this effect. In fact, 203 women with recurrent vaginal yeast infections who used echinacea for 10 weeks straight showed no decrease in measured indicators of immunity,[15] and some measures improved over the period.

In Australia, medical professionals frequently give echinacea in high doses for many months or even more than a year; no adverse effects have been reported.[16]

Another concern over long-term use of echinacea is that adverse side effects of medications often do not show up until the treatments have been used for a long time. In the case of drugs, there are established formal reporting systems intended to catch even complications that occur only rarely. However, the United States has no such formal system in place for herbs. Germany does have a reporting system of this type, but its requirements are less stringent than what is standard for drugs. Thus, although echinacea doesn't seem to produce any long-term adverse effects, it's difficult to be absolutely sure.

Is Echinacea Safe During Pregnancy and While Nursing?

Pregnancy and nursing present special concerns. Since echinacea has not been formally studied in pregnant or nursing women, we can't definitely know whether it is safe. In medicine, the standard practice is to *not* use medications in pregnant or nursing women unless (1) strong evidence establishes that the medicines are safe, or (2) the need for medication is so strong that the benefits appear to outweigh the risks. Herbalists, however, frequently recommend echinacea for occasional use in pregnant women, particularly after the first trimester, when the danger of birth defects is much less. If you choose to take echinacea while pregnant or nursing, keep in mind that the practice has not been scientifically proven to be safe.

Is Echinacea Safe for Children?

As for pregnant and nursing women, special caution appears sensible when considering the use of any treatment in young children. There have not been any studies of oral echinacea in children. However, oral echinacea should be even safer than injected echinacea, and more than 550 children with whooping cough ranging in age from infancy to 14 years old were given injected echinacea extract in German studies conducted since the 1950s.[17] No significant adverse effects were reported other than occasional modest rise in temperature, believed to be a sign of immune system activation. Similar results were seen in a report on the treatment of more than 500 children with tuberculosis.

Many practitioners give children echinacea for colds, and many echinacea preparations are intended for children. The dose is typically reduced according to the relative weight of the child as compared to an adult. While this practice has not been scientifically proven to be safe, practitioners who prescribe the herb have reported no problems.

Is Echinacea Safe for Those with Severe Liver or Kidney Disease?

Because the body eliminates most substances through the liver or kidneys, people with diseases in these organs should exercise special caution when using drugs. Whether similar precautions apply to echinacea use has not been determined.

Drug Interactions

No drug interactions are known to occur with echinacea. This doesn't mean they can't happen, just that none have been documented.

Echinacea: Not for Serious Infections

In addition to the diseases mentioned above, for which you should use echinacea cautiously, echinacea should not be used in certain instances. Echinacea is not a suitable substitute for appropriate drugs, such as antibiotics, in treating dangerous infections. In particular, do not rely on echinacea for the treatment of strep throat. If you feel you may be suffering from something worse than a common cold or flu, consult your physician. People in high-risk groups, as described in chapter 3, should not rely on echinacea as a substitute for flu vaccine or flu medications.

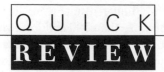

- Echinacea causes few side effects, although some people report general symptoms such as upset stomach or allergic reactions.

- No serious adverse effects due to echinacea use have been reported. For that reason, German physicians regard it as a nontoxic herb. However, the safety of echinacea has not been comprehensively studied using a formal research process.

- On a theoretical basis, some authorities recommend against using echinacea if you have an autoimmune disease, leukemia, AIDS, or tuberculosis. Others warn against using it for more than 8 weeks. However, no reliable evidence suggests that echinacea poses any risk in these circumstances.

- The safety of echinacea for children and pregnant or nursing women has not been scientifically established, although it is widely used in those groups.

CHAPTER
EIGHT

Other Herbs
for Colds
and Flus

E chinacea may help reduce the symptoms and duration of a cold, and perhaps even stop it entirely, but it certainly doesn't always work. Where do we go if echinacea doesn't work? There are a few other options offered by alternative medicine, some of which we'll look at in this chapter.

While these less familiar (at least in North America) herbal options have not been extensively researched, there is some evidence to support the use of at least a few of them. The herb andrographis, sometimes called "Indian echinacea" probably has the best evidence to its credit. But we'll begin by discussing ginseng and related herbs, because they are said to produce that most important of all possible benefits: improving immunity overall and thereby preventing colds from even starting. As we discussed in chapter 5, echinacea does not seem to have this capacity to any significant extent.

Ginseng: Said to Be an "Adaptogen"

This ancient Chinese herb was the first herb Russian scientist Dr. Israel I. Brekhman identified as an *adaptogen*. Brekhman coined the term to denote herbs that are supposed to be able to help the body resist stress of any type and return it to a state of "balance." Dr. Brekhman and his colleagues stated that for an herb to qualify as an adaptogen, it must meet three conditions:

- effectively treat a wide variety of illnesses
- help the individual's body return to a state of balance, no matter what is causing the imbalance, and
- cause no side effects

If there really were such a thing as an adaptogen, it would be a wonderful treatment to have. Unfortunately, the evidence that ginseng or any other herb really possesses these marvelous properties remains quite incomplete. We do have some fairly good evidence that ginseng may stimulate the immune system, however.

There is fairly good evidence that ginseng may stimulate the immune system.

Three different herbs are commonly called ginseng: *Panax ginseng* (Asian ginseng), *Panax quinquifolius* (American ginseng), and *Eleutherococcus senticosus* (Russian or Siberian "ginseng"). In fact, *Eleutherococcus* isn't in the ginseng family at all, but Dr. Brekhman believed that this herb possessed substantially similar properties and proposed it as a much less expensive alternative.

Asian ginseng grows in northern China, Korea, and Russia. The root of the plant is used for medicinal preparations (see figure 4). Traditionally, Asian ginseng was

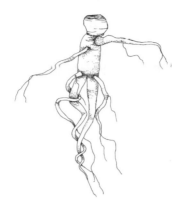

Figure 4. *Asian ginseng root* (Panax ginseng)

used as a "tonic" for the whole body or for specific organs such as the lungs. The traditional concept of a "tonic" indicates a substance that strengthens the body.

High-quality Asian ginseng root can command up to $8,000 per pound, partially because it must be grown and tended for at least five years before it can be harvested. Because of the high price of Asian ginseng, many products on the market that claim to contain this costly herb actually contain very little, or even none at all. Russian

High-quality Asian ginseng root can command up to $8,000 per pound.

"ginseng" (*Eleutherococcus*), on the other hand, is much easier to cultivate and does not command such a high price, so it is often substituted in formulas.

Most of the scientific research on ginseng was performed in the former Soviet Union and does not remotely reach current scientific standards. However, Asian,

Panax ginseng: The Chinese Perspective

While ginseng was popularized in the West by the Russian scientist Dr. Israel I. Brekhman, it was originally developed for use as a medicinal herb in China. Interestingly, the Chinese understanding of ginseng differs considerably from the way Brekhman understood it. To explain the difference, we need to first take a small detour and introduce the principles of Chinese medicine.

According to this ancient system of healing, illness is primarily caused by loss of balance between major body systems. Treatment does not focus on treating disease; rather, it aims at restoring balance in a fundamentally individualized way.

Consider the following analogy: If a person is leaning toward the left and in danger of toppling over, a gentle nudge applied toward the right will prevent a fall. However, if a person is leaning to the right, force must be applied toward the

European, and American research teams have performed higher-quality studies.

What Is Ginseng Used for Today?

Evidence suggests that ginseng may be able to increase the activity of the immune system. Test tube studies have found that ginseng, like echinacea, may increase white blood cell activity.[1]

More important, a recent double-blind study of 227 people in Italy found positive results with ginseng.[2] The researchers wanted to examine whether a standardized extract of ginseng root would improve immune responses to a flu vaccine.

left. No single intervention, no one direction of nudging, will stop everyone from falling—It all depends on the particular case.

The same is true of the improvements in balance that promote healing. There is no "one size fits all" in Chinese medical theory. What is good for one person is bad for another, because each person's needs are unique.

Thus according to the Chinese tradition, ginseng is only good for certain people and under certain conditions: It is useful for people who need precisely the "shove" that ginseng provides. According to theory, if the wrong people take ginseng, rather than improving their health, the herb will actually make them sicker! This directly contradicts Brekhman's adaptogen concept, which says that ginseng will help no matter what way you are out of balance.

The researchers gave people either placebo or 100 mg of standardized ginseng extract daily for 12 weeks. Everyone received a flu vaccination a month into the study. After the vaccine, the placebo group reported 42 cases of colds or flus but the treated group reported only 15 cases of colds or flus, a difference that was statistically significant (see figure 5). In addition, the treated group had a significantly greater rise in antibodies that fight influenza.

Researchers noted a few minor adverse effects during the study, the most prominent of which was insomnia. They also followed 24 laboratory-measured "safety parameters" and noted no significant difference between the

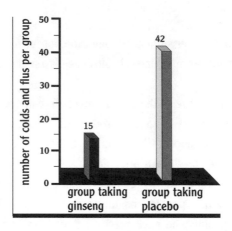

Figure 5. *Double-blind study shows ginseng reduced the number of colds and flus* (See et al., 1997)

two groups for these. Their conclusion was that ginseng improved immune response while having minimal adverse effects.

Dosage

Most of the studies of ginseng used products containing standardized ginseng extracts. Although we don't know how to tell if one form of ginseng is more effective than another based on this standardization, such extracts do ensure that you're buying the plant you think you are buying and not paying a premium price for Asian ginseng but getting the less expensive *Eleutherococcus*. (This, of course, assumes that the manufacturer honestly reports the results of standardized testing, which is not required by U.S. regulatory authorities.)

- *Panax ginseng:* The typical dose is 100 to 200 mg of standardized ginseng extract (standardized to 4 to 7%

ginsenosides) daily. This will probably be in capsule or tablet form. You will need to take up to 1 to 2 g per day (capsules or tablets) or 2 to 3 ml (tincture) of nonstandardized extracts, which are not as powerful.

- *Eleutherococcus:* 300 to 400 mg per day of standardized solid extract (standardized on eleutherosides B and E), or 4 to 5 ml of tincture twice per day. If you are taking a dried, nonstandardized product (powdered root or rhizome), take 2 to 3 g per day.

Traditionally, herbalists recommended taking ginseng for 6 to 8 weeks, then taking a break of 1 to 2 weeks before starting to take it again.[2] No studies, however, support the need for taking ginseng in this off and on way.

Safety Issues

The various forms of ginseng appear to be non-toxic, both in the short and long term, according to the results of studies in mice, rats, chickens, and dwarf pigs. Ginseng also does not seem to be carcinogenic.[3]

Reported side effects are rare. The double-blind Italian study found few side effects other than occasional insomnia,[4] and others report menstrual abnormalities and/or breast tenderness from women taking Asian ginseng.[5] Unconfirmed reports suggest that very high doses of ginseng (greater than 10 times the normal dose) can raise blood pressure, increase heart rate, and possibly cause other significant effects. Whether some of these cases were actually caused by caffeine mixed in with ginseng remains unclear, but we know that some manufacturers have at times added caffeine to their ginseng products (and "forgotten" to put it on the labels). Ginseng allergy can also occur, as can allergy to any other substance. Although allergic reactions would be extremely uncommon, highly allergic individuals should introduce ginseng into their lives cautiously just in case.

In 1979, an article published in the *Journal of the American Medical Association* claimed that people can become addicted to ginseng and develop blood pressure elevation, nervousness, sleeplessness, diarrhea, and hypersexuality. This report has since been thoroughly discredited and should no longer be taken seriously.[6,7]

Clinicians who use ashwaganda often report that it is as effective as ginseng, but gentler in action.

Safety in young children, pregnant or nursing women, or those with severe liver or kidney disease has not been established.

There are no definite drug interactions known to occur with ginseng. However, there has been one recent report of Siberian ginseng *(Eleuthrococcus)* apparently causing a potentially dangerous increase in blood levels of digoxin, a drug to regulate heart rhythm.[8]

Another report cited an interaction between ginseng and an MAO inhibitor drug, which is one of a class of drugs used for depression,[9] but the result could have been due to possible adulteration with caffeine.

Ashwaganda: "Indian Ginseng"

Its botanical name is *Withania somniferum,* but ashwaganda is sometimes called "Indian ginseng." This is because, in the Ayurvedic medical system (from India), ashwaganda is often used in much the same way the Asians use ginseng, as a tonic herb.

What Is Ashwaganda Used for Today?

Like ginseng, ashwaganda is said to increase the body's resistance to infection when it is taken for an extended period of time. Clinicians who use ashwaganda often report that it is as effective as ginseng, but gentler in action. However, we have almost no scientific evidence to which we can turn.

Researchers in one study fed ashwaganda to mice with aspergilliosis infections.[10] Mice that were given the herb survived longer than mice that did not get it. The researchers believed these results were due to improvements in some aspects of immune system activity, including phagocytosis (the ingesting of antigens by certain white blood cells).

Traditionally, maitake was used as a tonic to promote wellness and energy, to fight infections, and to adapt to stress.

Dosage

A typical dose of ashwaganda is 1 teaspoon of powder boiled in water or milk taken twice a day.

Safety Issues

Ashwaganda appears safe in normal doses, although only limited safety studies have been done. Due to the uncertainties, it should not be used by young children, pregnant or lactating women, or those with serious liver or kidney disease.

Maitake: Revered, but Has Little Science Behind It

Maitake is a medicinal mushroom, originally growing wild in the mountains of northeastern Japan and now cultivated by Japanese farmers.

What Is Maitake Used for Today?

Maitake is used both as a food (it tastes good) and as a medicinal herb. It has had almost magical powers attributed to it. Traditionally, maitake was used as a tonic to promote wellness and energy, to fight infections, and to adapt to stress. On this basis, some modern herbalists have decided that maitake must be an adaptogen. Limited research is now being done on a part of maitake called polysaccharides, which researchers speculate may be useful in treating diabetes,[11] hypertension,[12] and high cholesterol.[13,14,15]

At this time, we have no definitive evidence that maitake is effective.

In addition, it has been suggested that maitake's polysaccharides may stimulate immune system activity. As with echinacea, we are not sure that this is true (see chapter 5 for a discussion of the polysaccharides in echinacea). At this time, we have no definitive studies. Still, without waiting for evidence, many practitioners recommend maitake as an immune system stimulant.

Dosage

Maitake can be used in food or made into a tea, or if you purchase it in tablet or capsule form, you can take a dose of 3 to 7 g daily.

Safety Issues

While the herb is widely believed to be safe, formal safety studies of maitake have not yet been conducted. Safety in young children, pregnant or nursing women, or those with severe liver or kidney disease has not been established.

Other Adaptogens

The Brazilian herb *suma*, the Russian herb *rodiola*, and a Japanese fungus called *reishi mushroom* are also said to be adaptogens.

Other Possible
Herbal Immune Stimulants

Besides echinacea and the herbs considered adaptogens, there are other herbs that some believe can kick-start the immune system. However, none has been researched rigorously.

Andrographis: "Indian Echinacea"
Has Some Scientific Evidence

Andrographis is a shrub found throughout India and other Asian countries. It has been used historically in epidemics, including the Indian flu epidemic in 1919, where andrographis was credited with saving lives and stopping the spread of the disease.[16]

What Is Andrographis Used for Today?

Andrographis has recently gained a reputation as "Indian echinacea" because it is believed to work similarly. Over the last decade, it has become popular in Scandinavia as a treatment for colds. A few well-designed double-blind studies that found andrographis to be effective have recently been published in English. The evidence suggests that andrographis reduces the symptoms and duration of colds.

One study involved 50 people with colds given either andrographis or placebo. The results showed that 55% of the treated participants reported that their colds were less intense than usual, while only 19% of those in the placebo group stated this. The treated group averaged only 0.2

days of sick leave, while the untreated patients averaged 1 full day of sick leave. Finally, 75% of the treated patients

were well after 5 days, compared to less than 40% in the placebo group.[17]

Andrographis is popular in Scandinavia as a treatment for colds.

A study of 59 people from 18 to 60 years old found similar results.[18] Furthermore, a randomized, double-blind study involving 152 adults compared the effectiveness of andrographis (in doses of 3 g per day or 6 g per day, for 7 days) to acetaminophen for sore throat and fever. The higher dose of andrographis decreased symptoms of fever and throat pain, as did acetaminophen, while the lower dose of andrographis (3 g) did not. There were no significant side effects in either group.[19]

Although much more research remains to be performed, these results are quite promising.

Dosage

A typical dose of andrographis is 400 mg 3 times a day. Doses as high as 1,000 to 2,000 mg have been used in some studies. Andrographis is typically standardized to its content of andrographolide, usually 4 to 6% in commercial products. However, we don't know if this is important, and the 59-person study above used a product standardized to 4% andrographolides.

Safety Issues

No significant adverse effects have been reported in human studies of andrographis. The 59-person study mentioned earlier asked participants to report side effects, in addition to monitoring lab tests for liver function, complete blood counts, kidney function, and some other laboratory measures of toxicity. All of their tests came back within normal limits for both the placebo and the andrographis group.[20] However, full formal safety studies have not been completed. For this reason, the herb is not recommended for young children, pregnant or nursing women, or those with severe liver or kidney disease.

Some studies have raised concerns that andrographis may impair fertility. One study showed that male rats became infertile when fed 20 mg of andrographis powder per day.[21] In this case, the rats stopped producing sperm and exhibited physical changes in some of the testicular cells involved in sperm production. Researchers also detected evidence of degeneration of structures in the testicles. However, another study showed no evidence of testicular toxicity in male rats that were given up to 1 g per kilogram of body weight per day for 60 days, so this issue remains unclear.[22]

> **The evidence suggests that andrographis reduces the symptoms and duration of colds.**

One group of female mice also did not fare well on andrographis.[23] When fed 2 g per kilogram of body weight daily for 6 weeks (a dose thousands of times higher than the usual human dose), all female mice failed to get pregnant when mated with males of proven fertility. Meanwhile, of the control females, 95.2% got pregnant when mated with a similar group of male mice.

While andrographis is probably not a useful form of birth control, these animal studies warrant further investigation.

Elderberry: A Traditional Native American Herb That May Be Helpful for Flus

Native Americans used tea made from elderberry flowers to treat respiratory infections. They also used the leaves and flowers in poultices applied to wounds, and the bark, suitably aged, as a laxative.

What Is Elderberry Used for Today?

Elderberry flowers are commonly recommended to be taken at the onset of a cold or flu to avert a full-scale infection. A preliminary double-blind study has backed up this recommendation by finding that a standardized elderberry extract can significantly reduce the length and severity of flu symptoms.[24]

Preliminary evidence suggests that elderberry can reduce the length and severity of flu symptoms.

It has been suggested that elderberry works by inhibiting flu viruses, but much remains to be discovered.

Dosage

Elderberry-flower tea is made by steeping 3 to 5 g of dried flowers in 1 cup of boiling water for 10 to 15 minutes. A typical dose is 1 cup 3 times daily. Standardized extracts should be taken according to the directions on the product's label.

Safety Issues

Elderberry flowers are generally regarded as safe. Side effects are rare and consist primarily of occasional mild gastrointestinal distress or allergic reactions.

Nonetheless, safety in young children, pregnant or nursing women, or those with severe liver or kidney disease is not established.

Astragalus: A Traditional Chinese Herb with Little Scientific Support

Astragalus has been used by Chinese herbalists for centuries. Like all traditional Chinese herbs, astragalus was always combined with other herbs in a formula tailored to the individual. Herb combinations containing astragalus were used for a variety of purposes, including protecting against colds.

What Is Astragalus Used for Today?

Based on its use in traditional Chinese medicine, Western herbalists decided that astragalus must boost the immune system and began to use it much like echinacea. However, no reliable scientific evidence backs up this use.

Only a few studies exist. In one study, astragalus was given to mice whose immune system activity was decreased. After they were given astragalus, their cell-mediated immunity improved. These mice made more interferon and t-cells, and their macrophages were more active.[25]

There is no reliable scientific evidence for the use of astragalus.

While this observation suggests that astragalus may stimulate an immune system that has been weakened, it does not tell us anything definitive about astragalus's possible effects on the normal human immune system, nor does it give us any clues about whether astragalus can prevent colds or flus.

Dosage

A typical daily dose of astragalus is 9 to 30 g of dried root, boiled in water. Alcohol- and water-extracts of astragalus are available as well. These should be taken according to the instructions you'll find on the label. According to traditional Chinese medicine, you should use astragalus only when you are well, to prevent disease. Supposedly the herb will "drive the illness deeper" if you take it when you are sick.

Safety Issues

Comprehensive safety studies of astragalus have not been performed, but neither have any serious adverse effects been reported. Side effects also appear to be rare, usually limited to mild stomach upset or allergic reactions. The herb's safety has not yet been established for young children, pregnant or nursing women, or those with severe liver or kidney disease.

Garlic: Famous, but There's No Evidence That It's Effective

Garlic is an extremely popular herb, odor notwithstanding. Culinary uses are extremely common, and most cooks would not consider running out of garlic in their kitchens. It's becoming popular in the medicine cabinet, too.

What Is Garlic Used for Today?

Its most common use today (aside from cooking, of course) is for reducing cholesterol. (For more information, see *The Natural Pharmacist Guide to Garlic and Cholesterol.*) In addition, studies show that garlic decreases platelet aggregation (making it a "blood thinner")

A Bulb of Garlic . . .

Garlic has quite a reputation. From warding off vampires to eliminating parasites to lowering cholesterol, this herb has been used medicinally for centuries. It was even thought at one time to possess magical powers. Historically, garlic has been used for the following:

headaches	parasites	prevention
high blood pressure	infections,	of plague
endurance	especially	cough
and strength	wounds	fever
improvement	earaches	any stomach
heart disease	hemlock and	problems
and high blood	henbane	
pressure	poisoning	
tumors	acne	

and possibly lowers blood pressure, which may translate to additional benefits for the heart.[26,27] It is also being researched for possible benefits in preventing cancer.[28,29]

Garlic also has a traditional reputation for preventing colds and warding off vampires. However, these uses are not yet supported by any reliable evidence (especially the vampire part!).

One report stated that garlic can improve some aspects of immune system activity, including white blood cell count, natural killer cell activity, and phagocytosis.[30] However, as we have mentioned many times, this evidence does not really establish that eating garlic will improve immunity.

Garlic does have antibiotic properties that do not pertain to immunity. Unfortunately, garlic is only a topical

antibiotic, meaning that it kills bacteria when it touches them (like Bacitracin, bleach, and iodine). It does not appear that garlic works like penicillin as a whole-body antibiotic if you take it by mouth.

There is no reliable evidence that garlic can prevent colds.

Dosage

Many herbalists who recommend garlic for colds believe that only raw garlic is effective, and that powdered garlic is better for lowering cholesterol. For fresh garlic, you could take one clove every few hours (raw is preferred); for powdered garlic in capsules, take 1 to 2 capsules every few hours. The odor alone may scare the illness away, and if it doesn't, it will probably keep all your contagious co-workers from hanging around and infecting you.

Safety Issues

Because garlic is widely consumed as a food, it is generally believed to be safe. However, because garlic decreases

blood clotting, you should not combine it with prescription blood thinners such as Coumadin (warfarin). Excessive garlic intake can also cause stomach distress, nervousness, gas, and bloating.

You should not combine garlic with prescription blood thinners.

Goldenseal: A Misrepresented Herb

No discussion of herbal immune stimulants would be complete without mentioning goldenseal, though not for the reasons you might think. An extremely popular herb, it is widely used in North America, but usually for the wrong reasons. Goldenseal does appear to be a topical antibiotic, like garlic. However, despite the fact that echinacea/goldenseal combinations are widely sold for treatment of the common cold, this combination doesn't really make any sense.[31] No evidence supports the idea that goldenseal raises immunity or kills

There is no evidence that goldenseal offers any benefits when taken at the onset of a cold.

the cold virus. Furthermore, traditional herbalists do not recommend using goldenseal at the onset of a cold. Goldenseal was (and is) sometimes used later during a cold to loosen mucus congestion.

Since goldenseal is currently an endangered plant, you should avoid using it for colds and flus; it really isn't appropriate and you may contribute to the loss of this plant species.

Another characteristic incorrectly assigned to goldenseal is that it can block a positive drug test. This mistaken belief has led to enormous sales of the herb, and probably to numerous problems with the law since it doesn't work for that purpose.

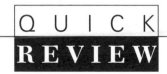

QUICK REVIEW

- Please refer to the chapter for safety information on these herbs.

- A group of herbs called adaptogens are widely believed to strengthen immunity. Ginseng is the most famous herb of this type, and the only one with any real scientific evidence behind it.

  For *Panax ginseng:* The typical dose is 100 to 200 mg of standardized ginseng extract (standardized to 4 to 7% ginsenosides) daily. This will probably be in capsule or tablet form. You will need to take up to 1 to 2 g per day (capsules or tablets) or 2 to 3 ml (tincture) of nonstandardized extracts, which are not as powerful.

  For *Eleutherococcus* ("Siberian ginseng"): 300 to 400 mg per day of standardized solid extract (standardized on eleutherosides B and E), or 4 to 5 ml of tincture twice per day. If you are taking a dried, nonstandardized product (powdered root or rhizome), take 2 to 3 g per day.

  Traditionally, herbalists recommended taking ginseng for 6 to 8 weeks, then taking a break of 1 to 2 weeks before starting to take it again.

  Other herbs in the adaptogen category said to improve immunity include ashawaganda, maitake, suma, rodiola, and reishi.

- The Indian herb andrographis is widely used in Scandinavia as a treatment for colds. It appears to reduce the symptoms and duration of colds. A typical dose of andrographis is 400 mg 3 times a day, taken with lots of liquids at mealtimes. Andrographis is typically standardized to its andrographolide content, usually 4 to 6% in commercial products.

- The traditional Native American herb elderberry may reduce the duration and severity of flu symptoms. Follow the label instructions for dosage recommendations.

- Although there is practically no scientific evidence, both garlic and the Chinese herb astragalus are said to increase immunity.

- Finally, despite its widespread fame as an "immune stimulant," goldenseal has neither tradition nor science to support its use in treating colds. Since goldenseal is endangered, please choose more appropriate herbs.

Nutrition for a Healthy Immune System

Many vitamins and minerals promote the normal functions of your immune system. We discussed them a bit in chapter 2 but will revisit them here. You need adequate amounts of these nutrients for your immune system to function optimally, though there is little convincing research showing that supplementation is necessary or beneficial in most cases.

Zinc

Although the mineral zinc is present in very small amounts in the body, it helps many parts of your body function. Among the systems that require adequate zinc is the immune system; white blood cells in particular require the mineral. Found in seafood, tofu, black-eyed peas, and wheat germ, zinc is a mineral many people in North America don't eat enough of, even though we don't need a lot.

Zinc deficiency decreases the functioning of t-cells and macrophages.[1,2] This means that maintaining adequate zinc in your diet is important. One study found that nursing home patients given supplements of zinc and selenium developed fewer colds. As many as two-thirds of the participants were deficient in these nutrients to begin with.[3]

Besides taking zinc for nutritional purposes, there is another popular way to use it: sucking on zinc lozenges to help prevent colds. However, the evidence for this method is mixed. Studies show both positive and negative results. It appears that the precise chemical form of zinc, along with sweeteners and other additives in the zinc lozenge, makes a big difference in its effectiveness. Nonetheless, there have even been contradictory results between studies using the same form of zinc.

A recent randomized, double-blind study involving 100 hospital employees found that zinc gluconate lozenges did decrease the severity and duration of the common cold. Participants used lozenges with 13.3 mg of zinc gluconate (or placebo) every 2 hours (while they were awake) for the duration of their colds.[4] The treated group had statistically significant reductions in cough, headache, hoarseness, nasal congestion, runny nose, and sore throat (see figure 6). In addition, their colds lasted an average of 4.4 days, significantly less than the 7.6 days' duration of colds for the placebo group.

Zinc gluconate (lozenges) may be beneficial for colds when started within 48 hours.

The symptoms not significantly affected by the zinc were fever, muscle aches, scratchy throat, and sneezing. The only side effect noted was mild nausea.

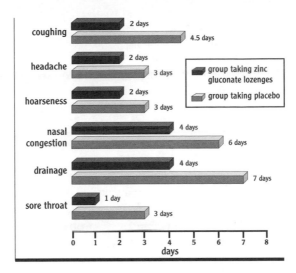

Figure 6. *Double-blind study shows zinc lozenges reduced the number of days participants experienced cold symptoms* (Mossad, et al., 1996)

However, another recent zinc gluconate lozenge study, which involved children, does not show such good results.[5] In this case, children in grades 1 through 6 were given 10 mg of zinc gluconate 5 times per day, and children in grades 7 through 12 were given 10 mg 6 times per day. There was no evidence that the zinc reduced the duration or severity of colds in these children, indicating that zinc gluconate lozenges might not be useful for childhood colds, though they do appear to be useful for adults. There is no good explanation for this failure, as the type of zinc used was identical to what was used in the study above.

Putting all the evidence together, zinc gluconate may be beneficial for colds when started within 48 hours of the onset and used regularly, but further research is necessary to iron out the contradictory reports.[6]

Dosage

To treat common colds, take zinc gluconate in lozenge form at a dose of 15 mg every 2 hours. The minimum effective dose studied was 13.3 mg every 2 hours.[7] There is no evidence that taking more will increase effectiveness. Most zinc lozenges contain from 10 to 15 mg per lozenge.

Research suggests that zinc gluconate sweetened with glycine is the best form of zinc for colds.

Zinc lozenges work best when started as soon as possible after the onset of a cold and when taken every 2 hours (while you're awake). The lozenge must be dissolved in your mouth because it probably works by directly killing viruses. Do not continue the zinc lozenge treatment for more than a week, because excess zinc is toxic (see Safety Issues).

Research suggests that zinc gluconate is the only form that you should use, so don't use zinc sulfate or other zinc compounds. Zinc lozenges are usually sweetened or otherwise flavored to disguise the taste, but additives like citric acid, sorbitol, and mannitol may bind the zinc ions in your mouth and make it impossible for them to kill the viruses in your throat.[8,9] A substance called glycine appears to be okay as a sweetener.

Safety Issues

Excessive doses of zinc over many months can be toxic.[10,11] However, when zinc is taken at the recommended dosage and only for the duration of the cold, it appears to be completely safe.

And You Thought You Got
That Cold at Work . . .

Everyone knows that you feel better when you have friends, family, and a strong sense of belonging to a community. Now there is even research to support this.[12] A 1997 study examined the theory that people with more diverse social ties resist infections better than those with fewer relationships. The researchers looked at social ties, including those with spouse, parent, friend, workmate, and member of a social group, and studied susceptibility to colds among the 276 participants. They found that people with more types of social ties got fewer colds than did those with fewer social relationships. The people with the fewest ties (from one to three) were 4.2 times more likely to catch cold than were those with more than six social ties.

Vitamin C

A great deal of research has focused on the functions of vitamin C. We know, for example, that it is an important antioxidant. There is little evidence that vitamin C can prevent colds, but it does appear to help make them less severe. As everyone knows, vitamin C is found in citrus fruit, but it is also in broccoli, red peppers, strawberries, brussels sprouts, parsley, and currants.

Research has not shown, contrary to popular belief, that taking vitamin C prevents colds in general. There is, however, some evidence that it can decrease the incidence of colds in people who don't get much vitamin C from their diet.[13] It also seems to be helpful in preventing the colds that athletes frequently develop after running a marathon.[14,15] Also, substantial evidence shows that vitamin C does modestly decrease the severity and possibly the duration of colds.[16,17]

Dosage

During a cold, you can take vitamin C at doses of 500 to 1,000 mg 3 times a day. If you notice any stomach upset, especially diarrhea, cut back by 250 mg per dose. This diarrhea is a sign that you've reached your "bowel tolerance" of vitamin C, and it means your body can't handle the amount you are taking. If your cold persists for more than a few days, you can increase your vitamin C dose by 500 mg per day after you have waited a couple of days at your bowel tolerance level. After a couple of days, your body should be able to handle the increased dose just fine.

Substantial evidence shows that vitamin C can modestly decrease the severity and possibly the duration of colds.

Vitamin C may be more effective if the same dose (500 to 1,000 mg 3 times per day) of mixed bioflavonoids is taken at the same time. Bioflavonoids are antioxidants that usually come with vitamin C in plants. For example, there are a lot of bioflavonoids in the white pulp inside the peel of citrus fruits.

Safety Issues

High doses of vitamin C can cause diarrhea, at least until you get used to taking it. Other than that, short-term use (at least) appears to be quite safe for most people. If you have severe kidney disease or suffer from gout or recurrent kidney stones, then you should take vitamin C only under a physician's supervision. In addition, high doses of vitamin C should not be taken with large doses of iron because the two can be toxic together.

Vitamin E

Of all the antioxidants, vitamin E is the one whose benefits in various diseases are most established. Good evidence suggests that regular use of vitamin E may reduce the risk of heart disease and some forms of cancer. One recent double-blind study suggests that vitamin E may offer immune benefits as well.

This study involved 88 adults over 65, all of whom were considered to be healthy and have normally functioning immune systems.[18] The subjects were given either placebo or vitamin E at various doses. The researchers then tested the subjects' immune responsiveness by giving them immunizations for hepatitis B, tetanus, diphtheria, and pneumonia. After the vaccinations, the researchers examined the level of immune response among the people taking the different levels of vitamin E or taking the placebo. They did so by using a test, like the TB test, called DTH. This test evaluates

A recent double-blind study strongly suggests that vitamin E can increase the activity of the immune system.

the overall strength of a person's cell-mediated immunity. The results show that the group taking 200 IU (international units) of vitamin E had significantly stronger responses on the DTH test. This strongly suggests that supplemental vitamin E can increase the activity of the immune system.

Dosage

The most common level of vitamin E supplementation is from 200 to 800 IU per day. The study above tested three dosages: 60 IU, 200 IU, and 800 IU per day. The researchers noted that the best effect was observed at 200 IU daily, and that 800 IU per day did not produce significantly better results. Based on this, we would recommend taking 200 IU of vitamin E daily.

Safety Issues

Vitamin E is believed to be very safe.[19] However, vitamin E slightly thins the blood, so it should not be combined with drugs such as Coumadin (warfarin) except on a physician's advice.

Dairy Culprit

Many people report that milk and dairy products appear to increase mucus congestion and lead to colds although no scientific evidence is available to support this. Practitioners of many schools of alternative medicine, naturopaths, nutritionists, and Chinese medicine practitioners agree. Conventional physicians, particularly pediatricians, often also share this view. These health-care professionals recommend that you avoid dairy products when you have cold or flu. This treatment seems to be quite effective for a many, but not all, people. To use this method to prevent colds, you have to quit using milk products for some time, perhaps a month. Hard cheese is less problematic than milk, and yogurt and cottage cheese are somewhere in between. This is presumably because hard cheese has aged so long that most of the offending constituents have been "chewed up" by the fermenting bacteria.

One of my patients, Peter, had been getting more than his share of colds. I advised him to quit drinking milk. At first he was skeptical, but when he was fighting his third cold of the winter, he finally relented. He called me a few days later, surprised at the results. "I didn't expect any change," he told me, "but there really has been one. I mean, I still have a runny nose, but my head is a lot clearer and I'm sleeping better. It really has helped." Peter's results are representative of the usual results I see. I don't expect miracles from cutting out dairy products, but most people see enough benefit that they are willing to cut them out entirely while they have colds. Some people even limit their dairy intake all winter, convinced that it helps them have fewer colds.

Many health-care professionals recommend that you avoid dairy products when you have a cold or flu.

If you do stop eating dairy products for more than a couple of weeks, make sure you get calcium and vitamin D from another source. Several other foods provide these essential nutrients, or you can take calcium and vitamin D supplements and drink calcium-fortified orange juice, soy milk, or rice milk.

Other Food Sensitivities

Peter probably had an allergy or sensitivity to milk. Many alternative practitioners feel that reactions to foods play a part in our daily susceptibility to illness, as well as to other conditions. The theory is that you may have a low-level intolerance for certain foods, perhaps due to a mild food

Food Sensitivities

Many alternative practitioners feel that food sensitivities play a part in our daily susceptibility to illness, as well as to other conditions. The theory is that you may have a low-level sensitivity to certain foods, similar but not necessarily identical to an allergy. This sensitivity may cause enough disturbance to the body to increase susceptibility to infection.

Some individuals do appear to benefit from eliminating certain foods from their diets. Unfortunately, performing double-blind studies on diet is next to impossible (since it's obvious whether or not you're eating cheese, for example). For this reason, it's difficult to discover just what role, if any, food sensitivities play in health and illness. If you suspect that certain foods don't agree with you, you could try avoiding

allergy or something else. Repeated exposure to foods you're sensitive to may stress your body and make you more prone to infections.

Unfortunately, performing double-blind studies on diet is next to impossible (try to imagine not knowing whether you are drinking milkshakes!). Some individuals do, however, appear to benefit from eliminating certain foods from their diets.

If you are aware that certain foods don't agree with you, try avoiding them when you get your next cold to see whether you feel better. Some of the most common foods mentioned as problematic besides milk are wheat, sugar, and caffeine-containing foods.[20–24] You can also try eliminating these foods for a long period of time and see if it reduces the number of colds you develop.

them when you get your next cold to see whether you recover faster. Some foods people commonly mention as problematic include milk, sugar, coffee and other caffeine-containing foods, and wheat and some other grains.

Avoiding these foods for a week or two to see whether they affect your body poses little risk. If you restrict your diet for a long time, however, you may suffer from malnutrition. We have said, repeatedly, that malnutrition can decrease immunity, and eliminating too many foods can cause malnutrition. If you are interested in a major diet overhaul, see a physician who can help you make sure you are still getting enough of all the essential nutrients. This is especially important for children, whose growing bodies require excellent nutrition.

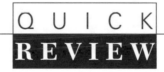

QUICK REVIEW

- Although the research evidence is somewhat contradictory, the use of zinc gluconate lozenges at the onset of a cold may reduce the severity and duration of the cold. The proper dose is 15 mg every 2 hours during the first few days of a cold. Do not take high doses of zinc for more than a week, as it can be toxic if overused.

- Vitamin C does not appear to prevent most colds but may reduce their duration and severity. When you get a cold, you can take vitamin C at doses of 500 to 1,000 mg 3 times a day. If you notice any stomach upset, especially diarrhea, cut back by 250 mg per dose.

- Vitamin E may offer immune benefits. The most common level of vitamin E supplementation is from 200 to 800 IU per day.

- Some people report that milk or other foods cause them to develop mucus, which may make their colds worse. Although no scientific evidence yet supports this, you may find it helpful to eliminate milk products and other foods to which you are sensitive, provided you take care to keep up your nutrition, especially making sure to get calcium and vitamin D from another source.

Putting It All Together

For your easy reference, this chapter contains a brief summary of key information contained in this book. Please refer to earlier chapters for more comprehensive information, including a detailed discussion of safety issues.

Echinacea is one of the most commonly used medicinal herbs in the world. Evidence suggests that it can reduce the severity and duration of a cold. It also may "abort" a cold if taken at the first sign of symptoms. However, long-term use of echinacea does not appear to offer much in the way of benefits.

Though echinacea and the other treatments mentioned below are safe for colds and flus, sometimes you need more help than they can provide. If you think you have developed a strep throat, sinus infection, or other complication of a cold or flu, see your doctor. You may need antibiotics, which can be lifesaving in some cases, though they are completely ineffective against the viruses that cause colds and flus.

Also, people at high risk for complications from influenza should get a flu vaccination at the beginning of flu season, and they may wish to use prescription flu medications such as rimantadine or amantadine.

There are three commonly used species of echinacea—*Echinacea angustifolia, Echinacea purpurea,* and *Echinacea pallida*. It is not clear which of these is best for treating colds and flus. The most widely available form is *E. purpurea*.

Echinacea is available in many forms, each with its own suggested dosage:

> *Dried root:* 0.5 to 1 g 3 times per day
> *Juice:* 2 to 3 ml (½ to ¾ teaspoon) 3 times per day
> *Tincture (1:5):* 2 to 4 ml (½ to 1 teaspoon) 3
>   times per day
> *Fluid extract (1:1):* 1 to 2 ml (¼ to ½ teaspoon)
>   3 times per day
> *Dry, powdered extract (standardized to 3.5% echinacoside):* 300 mg 3 times per day
> *Freeze-dried:* 1 to 2 capsules or tablets 3 times
>   per day

These dosage recommendations, however, are only approximations. When in doubt, consult a qualified health-care practitioner.

Echinacea appears to be non-toxic, and most people suffer no side effects from taking echinacea. Allergic reactions are practically the only side effects reported, and they are rare.

On a theoretical basis, some authorities recommend against using echinacea if you have an autoimmune disease, leukemia, tuberculosis, or AIDS. Others warn against using it for more than 8 weeks. However, no reliable evidence suggests that echinacea poses any risk in these circumstances.

There are no reports of echinacea/drug interactions or interactions between echinacea and other herbs or foods or any other substances.

Other Natural Treatments for Colds

A class of herbs called "adaptogens" is widely believed to strengthen immunity, although there is little research evidence. **Ginseng** is the most famous adaptogen, followed by **ashwaganda**, **maitake**, and others.

Traditionally, herbalists recommended taking ginseng for 6 to 8 weeks, then taking a break of 1 to 2 weeks before starting to take it again.

Two distinct herbs are called ginseng. Dosages are as follows:

Panax ginseng: The typical dose is 100 to 200 mg of standardized ginseng extract (standardized to 4 to 7% ginsenosides) daily.

Eleutherococcus ("Siberian ginseng"): 300 to 400 mg per day of standardized solid extract (standardized on eleutherosides B and E), or 4 to 5 ml of tincture twice per day. If you are taking a dried, non-standardized product (powdered root or rhizome), take 2 to 3 g per day.

Another herb you may wish to explore further is the Indian herb **andrographis**, widely used in Scandinavia as a treatment for colds. According to a few double-blind studies, it can reduce the symptoms and duration of colds. A typical dose of andrographis is ½ to 1 teaspoon 3 times a day, taken with lots of liquid at mealtimes.

Additional herbs sometimes recommended for colds include **elderberry, garlic,** and the Chinese herb **astragalus.**

Despite its widespread fame as an "immune stimulant," there is no evidence that the herb goldenseal produces any such benefit, and traditionally it was not used for this purpose.

Vitamins and Minerals

In addition to herbal remedies, some minerals (such as **zinc**) and vitamins (such as **vitamins C** and **E**) may be helpful for colds.

Although the research evidence is somewhat contradictory, the use of zinc gluconate lozenges at the onset of a cold may reduce the severity and duration of the cold. The proper dose is 15 mg every 2 hours during the first few days of a cold. Do not take high-dose zinc for more than a week, as it can be toxic if overused.

Vitamin C does not appear to prevent most colds but may reduce their duration and severity. When you get a cold, you can take vitamin C at dosages of 500 to 1,000 mg 3 times a day. If you notice any stomach upset, especially diarrhea, cut back by 250 mg per dose.

Vitamin E may offer immune benefits. The most common level of vitamin E supplementation is from 200 to 800 IU per day.

Notes

Chapter One

1. Snow JM. *Echinacea* (Moench) spp. Asteraceae. *The Protocol Journal of Botanical Medicine* 2(2): 18–24, 1997.

2. Snow JM, 1997.

3. Bauer R and Wagner H. Echinacea species as potential immunostimulatory drugs. *Econ Med Plant Res* 5: 253–321, 1991.

4. Bone K. Echinacea: What makes it work? *Altern Med Review* 2(2): 87–93, 1997.

5. Heinzer F, et al. Classification of the therapeutically used species of the genus Echinacea. *Pharm Acta Helv* 63(4–5): 132–136, 1988.

6. Snow JM, 1997.

7. Snow JM, 1997.

8. Snow JM, 1997.

9. Snow JM, 1997.

10. Bone K, 1997.

11. Facino R and Meffei M. Direct characterization of caffeoyl esters with antihyaluronidase activity in crude extracts from *Echinacea angustifolia* roots by fast atom bombardment tandem mass spectrometry. *Farmaco* 48(10): 1447–1461, 1993.

12. Becker H and Hsieh, WC. Cichoric acid and its derivatives from Echinacea species. *Z Naturforsch C: Biosci* 40C(7–8): 585–587, 1985.

13. Snow JM, 1997.

14. Bergner P. The healing power of echinacea and goldenseal. Rocklin, CA: Prima Publishing, 1997.

15. Snow JM, 1997.

16. Bone K, 1997.

17. Facino RM, et al., 1993.

18. Becker J and Hsieh WC, 1985.

19. Bone K, 1997.

20. Bergner P, 1997.

21. Schulz V, et al. Rational phytotherapy. New York: Springer-Verlag, 278, 1998.

Chapter Two

1. Bartok L. Bacterial endotoxins and nonspecific resistance. *Acta Microbiol Immunol Hung* 44(4): 361–5, 1997.

2. Sali A. Psychoneuroimmunology: fact or fiction? *Aust Fam Physician* (11): 1291–4, 1296–1299, 26 Nov 1997.

3. Harrison's principles of internal medicine, 14th ed. New York: McGraw-Hill, 1998.

4. Chandra RK. Nutrition and immunity: lessons from the past and new insights into the future. *Am J Clin Nutr* 53: 1087–1101, 1991. As cited in Werbach M. Nutritional influences on illness, 2nd ed. Tarzana, CA: Third Line Press, 1993.

5. Anderson R and Theron A. Effects of B-complex vitamins on cellular and humoral immune functions in vitro and in vivo. *Int J Vitam Nutr Res,* 24: 77–84, 1983. As cited in Werbach M, 1993.

6. Levy JA. Nutrition and the immune system, in Stiles DP, et al. *Basic and Clinical Immunology*, 4th ed. Los Altos, CA: Lange Medical Publications, 297–305, 1982. As cited in Werbach M, 1993.

7. Beisel WR. Single nutrients and immunity. *Am J Clin Nutr* 35: 417–468 (supplement), 1982. As cited in Werbach M, 1993.

8. Beisel WR, et al. Single-nutrient effects on immunologic functions. *JAMA* 245(1): 53–58, 1981. As cited in Werbach M, 1993.

9. Levy JA, 1982.

10. Chandra RK, 1983.

11. Chandra RK, 1983.

12. Pocino M, et al. Influence of oral administration of excess copper on the immune response. *Fundam Appl Toxicol* 16: 249–256, 1991. As cited in Werbach M, 1993.

Chapter Three

1. Taber's cyclopedic medical dictionary, 17th ed. Philadelphia: F. A. Davis Company, 1888, 1989.

Chapter Four

1. Harrison's principles of internal medicine, 14th ed. New York: McGraw-Hill, 1998.

Chapter Five

1. Schulz V, et al. Rational phytotherapy. New York: Springer-Verlag, 246, 1998.

2. Melchart D, et al. Immunomodulation with echinacea: a systematic review of controlled clinical trials. *Phytomed* 1: 245–254, 1994. Reported in Schulz V, et al. Rational phytotherapy. New York: Springer-Verlag, 1998: 276.

3. Dorn M. Milderung grippaler Effekte durch ein pflanzliches Immunstimulans. *Natur und Ganzheitsmedizin* 2: 314–319, 1989. Reported in Schulz V, et al., 1998: 276

4. Dorn M, et al. Placebo-controlled, double-blind study of *Echinaceae pallidae* radix in upper respiratory tract infections. *Complement Ther Med* 3: 40–42, 1997.

5. Braunig B, et al. *Echinacea purpurea* radix for strengthening the immune response in flu-like infections. *Zeitschrift für Phytotherapie* 13: 7–13, 1992. Translated by Shanti Coble and Christopher Hobbs, 1992.

6. Hoheisel O, et al. Echinagard treatment shortens the course of the common cold: A double-blind placebo-controlled clinical trial. *Eur J Clin Res* 9: 261–268, 1997.

7. Schoneberger D. The influence of immune-stimulating effects of pressed juice from *Echinacea purpurea* on the course and severity of colds. *Forum Immunol* 8: 2–12, 1992. Translated by Sigrid M Klein, 1993.

8. Melchart, D, et al. Echinacea root extracts for the prevention of upper respiratory tract infections: a double-blind, placebo-controlled randomized trial. *Arch Fam Med* 7: 541–545, 1998.

9. Melchart D, et al., 1994.

10. Jurcic K, et al. Zwei Probandenstudien zur Stimulierung durch Echinacea-Extrakt-haltige Praparate. *Zeitschrift für Phytotherapie* 10: 67–70, 1989. English summary and reported in Bone K. *Altern Med Rev* 2(6): 451–458, 1997.

11. Bauer R, et al. *Zeitschrift fur Phytotherapie* 10: 43, 1989. As cited in Bone K. *Altern Med Rev* 2(2): 87–93, 1997.

12. Volmel VT. Einfluss eines unspezifischen immunstimulans auf die phagozytose von erthrozyten und tusche durch das retikulohistiozytare system unterschiedlich alter, isolert perfundierter rattenlebern. *Arzneimittel-Forschung/Drug Res* 34: 691–695, 1984. As cited in Snow JM. Echinacea (Moench) Spp. Asteraceae. *The Protocol Journal of Botanical Medicine* 2(2): 18–24, 1997.

13. Bauer VR, et al. Immunologische in vivo und in vitro unterschungen mit echinacea-extrakten. *Arzneimittel-Forschung/Drug Res* 38: 276–281, 1988. As cited in Snow, pp. 18–24, 1997.

14. Gaisbauer M, et al. Untersuchungen zum einflub von echinacea purpurea moench auf die phagozytose von granulozyten mittels messung der chemilumineszenz. *Arzneimittel-Forschung/Drug Res* 40: 594–598, 1990. As cited in Snow, pp. 18–24, 1997.

15. Wagner H and Proksch A. An immunostimulating active principal from *Echinacea purpurea* Moench. *Z. Angew. Phytother* 2(5): 166–168, 1981.

16. Stimple M, et al. Macrophage activation and induction of macrophage cytotoxicity by purified polysaccharide fraction of the plant *Echinacea purpurea*. *Infect Immun* 46(3): 845–849, 1984.

17. Luettig B, et al. Macropohage activation by the polysaccharide arabinogalactan isolated from plant cell cultures of *Echinacea purpurea. J Nat Cancer Inst* 81(9): 669–675, 1989.

18. Coeugniet E and Kuhnhast R. Recurrent candidiasis: adjuvant immunotherapy with different formulations of Echinacin Æ *Therapiewoche* 36: 3352–3358, 1986.

19. Wagner H and Proksch A, 1981.

20. Stimple M, et al., 1984.

21. Luettig B, et al., 1989.

22. Bone K. Echinacea: what makes it work? *Altern Med Rev* 2(2): 87–93, 1997.

23. Bauer R, et al. Immunological in vivo and in vitro examinations of echinacea extracts. *Arzneimittel-Forschung* 38(2): 276–281, 1988.

24. Bauer R, et al., 1988.

25. Bone K, 1997.

26. Coeugniet E and Kuhnhast R, 1986.

27. Tubaro A, et al. Anti-inflammatory activity of a polysaccharidic fraction of *Echinacea angustifolia. J Pharm Pharmacol* 39(7): 567, 1987.

28. Muller-Jakic B, et al. In vitro inhibition of cyclooxygenase and 5-lipoxygenase by alkamides from *Echinacea* and *Achillea* species. *Planta Med* 60(1): 37, 1994.

29. Tragni E, et al. Antiinflammatory activity *of Echinacea angustifolia* fractions separated on the basis of molecular weight. *Pharmacol Res Commun* 20(Suppl 5): 87, 1988.

30. Busing KH. Inhibition of hyaluronidase by echinacin. *Arzneimittel-Forschung* 2: 467–469, 1952. As cited in Snow, pp. 18–24, 1997.

31. Busing KH. Hyaluronidase inhibition of some naturally occurring substances used in therapy. *Arzneimittel-Forschung* 5: 320–322, 1955. As cited in Snow, pp. 18–24, 1997.

Chapter Six

1. Hoheisel O, et al. Echinagard treatment shortens the course of the common cold: a double-blind, placebo-controlled clinical trial. *Eur J Clin Res*, 9: 261–268, 1997.

2. Braunig B, et al, 1992.

3. Dorn M. Milderung grippaler Infekte durch ein pflanzliches Immunstimulans. *Natur und Ganzheitsmedizin* 2: 314–319. Reported in Schulz V, et al. Rational phytotherapy, New York: Springer-Verlag, 276, 1998.

4. Dorn M, et al. Placebo-controlled, double-blind study of *Echinacea pallidae* radix in upper respiratory tract infections. *Complement Ther in Med* 5(1): 40–42, 1997.

5. Bauer R, et al. Immunological in vivo and in vitro examinations of echinacea extracts. *Arzneimittel-Forschung* 38(2): 276–281, 1988.

Chapter Seven

1. Mosby's 1998 nursing drug reference. St. Louis, MO: Mosby, 1998.

2. Parnham MJ. Benefit-risk assessment of the squeezed sap of the purple coneflower *(Echinacea purpurea)* for long-term oral immunostimulation. *Phytomedicine* 3(1): 95–102, 1996.

3. Parnham MJ, 1996.

4. Bone K. Echinacea: what makes it work? *Alt Med Review* 2(2): 87–93, 1997.

5. Parnham MJ, 1996.

6. Parnham MJ, 1996.

7. Mullins RJ. Echinacea-associated anaphylaxis. *Med J Australia* 168(4): 170–171, 1998.

8. Schulz V, et al. Rational phytotherapy. New York: Springer-Verlag, 276, 1998.

9. Mengs U, et al. Toxicity of *Echinacea purpurea:* Acute, subacute and genotoxicity studies. *Arzneimittel Forschung* 41(10): 1076–1081, 1991.

10. Bauer R and Wagner H. Echinacea species as potential im-

munostimulatory drugs. *Econ Med Plant Res* 5: 253–321, 1991. As cited in Snow JM. Echinacea (Moench) spp. Asteraccae. *The Protocol Journal of Botanical Medicine* 2(2): 18–24, 1997.

11. Bone K, 1997.

12. McLeod D. Case history of chronic lymphocytic leukemia. *Modern Phytotherapist* 2(3): 34–35, 1996. As cited in Bone K, 1997.

13. Bergner P. The healing power of echinacea and goldenseal. Rocklin, CA: Prima Publishing, 115–116, 1997.

14. Bergner P, 118, 1997.

15. Coeugniet E and Kuhnhast R. Recurrent candidiasis: adjuvant immunotherapy with different formulations of echinacin Æ *Therapiewoche* 36: 3352–3358, 1986. As reported in Phytotherapy Research Compendium from the Herb Research Foundation.

16. Bergner P, 119, 1997.

17. Parnham MJ, 1996.

Chapter Eight

1. See DM, ct al. In vitro effects of echinacea and ginseng on natural killer cells and antibody-dependent cell cytoxicity in healthy subjects and chronic fatigue syndrome or acquired immunodeficiency patients. *Immunopharmacol* 35: 3, 229–235, 1997.

2. Scaglione F, et al. Efficacy and safety of the standardised ginseng extract G115 for potentiating vaccination against the influenza syndrome and protecting against the common cold. *Drugs Exp Clin Res* 22(2): 65–72, 1996.

3. Shulz, V. Rational phytotherapy New York: Springer-Verlag, 272, 1998.

4. Scaglione F, et al., 1996.

5. Baldwin CA, et al. What pharmacists should know about ginseng. *Pharm J* 237: 583–610, 1986. Tyler V, 1994.

6 Tyler V. Herbs of choice. New York: Howorth Press, 1994.

7. Schulz V, et al., 1998.

8. McRae S. Elevated serum digoxin levels in a patient taking digoxin and Siberian ginseng. *CMAJ* 155(3): 293–295, 1996.

9. Jones BD, et al. Interaction of ginseng with phenelzine. *J Clin Psychopharmacol* 7: 201–202, 1987.

10. Dhuley JN. Therapeutic efficacy of Ashwagandha against experimental aspergillosis in mice. *Immunopharmacol Immunotoxicol* 20(1): 191–198, 1998.

11. Kubo K, et al. Anti-diabetic activity present in the fruit body of *Grifola frondosa* (Maitake). I. *Biol Pharm Bull* 17(8): 1106–1110, 1994.

12. Kabir Y, et al. Effect of shiitake *(Lentinus edodes)* and maitake *(Grifola frondosa)* mushrooms on blood pressure and plasma lipids of spontaneously hypertensive rats. *J Nutr Sci Vitaminol* (Tokyo), 33(5): 341–346, 1987.

13. Kubo K and Nanba H. The effect of maitake mushrooms on liver and serum lipids. *Altern Ther Health Med* 2(5): 62–66, 1996.

14. Kubo K and Nanba H. Anti-hyperliposis effect of maitake fruit body *(Grifola frondosa)*. I. *Biol Pharm Bull* 20(7): 781–785, 1997.

15. Kabir Y, et al., 1987.

16. Hancke J, et al. A double-blind study with a new monodrug Kan Jang: decrease of symptoms and improvements in the recovery from common colds. *Phytother Res* 9: 559–562, 1995.

17. Melchior J, et al. Controlled clinical study of standardized *Andrographis paniculata* extract in common cold: a pilot trial. *Phytomedicine* 34:314–318, 1996–1997.

18. Hancke J, et al., 1995.

19. Thamlikitkul V, et al. Efficacy of *Andrographis paniculata* (Nees) for pharyngotonsillitis in adults. *J Med Assoc Thai* 74(10): 437–442, 1991.

20. Hancke J, et al., 1995.

21. Akbarsha MA, et al. Antifertility effect of *Andrographis paniculata* (Nees) in male albino rat. *Indian J Exp Biol* 28(5): 421–426, 1990.

22. Burgos RA, et al. Testicular toxicity assessment of *Andrographis paniculata* dried extract in rats. *J Ethnopharmacol* 58(3): 219–224, 1997.

23. Zoha MS, et al. Antifertility effect of *Andrographis paniculata* in mice. *Bangladesh Med Res Counc Bull* 15(1): 34–37, 1989.

24. Zakay-Rones Z, et al. Inhibition of several strains of influenza virus and reduction of symptoms by an elderberry extract (*Sambucus nigra* L.) during an outbreak of influenza B Panama. *J Altern Complement Med* 1(4): 361–369, 1995.

25. Liang H, et al. The effect of astragalus polysaccharides (APS) on cell mediated immunity (CMI) in burned mice. *Chung Hua Cheng Hsing Shao Shang Wai Ko Tsa Chih* 10(2): 138–141, 1994.

26. Romano EL, et al. Effects of ajoene on lymphocyte and macrophage membrane-dependent functions. *Immunopharmacol Immunotoxicol* 19(1): 15–36, 1997.

27. Silagy CA, et al. A meta-analysis of the effect of garlic on blood pressure. *J Hypertens* 12(4): 463–468, 1994.

28. Sumiyoshi H. New pharmacological activities of garlic and its constituents. *Nippon Yakurigaku Zasshi* 110(Suppl 1): 93P–97P, 1997.

29. Steinmetz KA, et al. Vegetables, fruit and colon cancer in the Iowa Women's Health Study. A *J Epidemiol* 139(1): 1–13, 1994.

30. Sumiyoshi H, 1997.

31. Bergner, P. The healing power of echinacea and goldenseal. Rocklin, CA: Prima Publishing, 1997.

Chapter Nine

1. Harrison's principles of internal medicine, 14th ed. New York: McGraw-Hill, 1998.

2. Chandra RK. Trace element regulation of immunity and infection. *J Am Coll Nutr* 4(1): 5–16, 1985.

3. Girodon F, et al. Effect of micronutrient supplementation

on infection in institutionalized elderly subjects: a controlled trial. *Ann Nutr Metab* 41(2): 98–107, 1997.

4. Mossad SB, et al. Zinc gluconate lozenges for treating the common cold. A randomized, double-blind, placebo-controlled study. *Ann Intern Medicine* 125(2): 81–88, 1996.

5. Macknin ML, et al. Zinc gluconate for treating the common cold in children: a randomized controlled trial. *JAMA* 279(24): 1962–1967, 1988.

6. Marshall S. Zinc gluconate and the common cold. Review of randomized controlled trials. *Can Family Physician* 44: 1037–1042, 1998.

7. Marshall S, 1998.

8. Marshall S, 1998.

9. Macknin ML, et al., 1988.

10. Harrison's, 1998.

11. Lewis MR and Kokan L. Zinc gluconate: acute ingestion. *J Toxicol Clin Toxicol* 36(1–2): 99–101, 1998.

12. Cohen S, et al. Social ties and susceptibility to the common cold. *JAMA* 277(24): 1940–1944, 1997.

13. Hemila H. Vitamin C intake and susceptibility to the common cold. *BMJ* 77(1): 59–72, 1997.

14. Peters EM, et al. Vitamin C supplementation reduces the incidence of postrace symptoms of upper-respiratory-tract infection in ultramarathon runners. *Am J Clin Nutr* 57(2): 170–174, 1993.

15. Hemila H. Vitamin C and common cold incidence: a review of studies with subjects under heavy physical stress. *Int J Sports Med* 17(5): 379–383, 1996.

16. Hemila H. Vitamin C, the placebo effect, and the common cold: a case study of how preconceptions influence the analysis of results. *J Clin Epidemiol* 49(10): 1079–1084, 1996.

17. Hemila H. Vitamin C and the common cold. *Br J Nutr* 67: 3–16, 1992.

18. Meydani SM, et al. Vitamin E supplementation and in vivo immune response in healthy elderly subjects: A randomized controlled trial. *JAMA* 277: 1380–1386, 1997.

19. Harrison's, 1998.

20. Bernstein J, et al. Depression of lymphocyte transformation following oral glucose ingestion. *Am J Clin Nutr* 30: 613, 1977. As cited in Werbach M. Nutritional Influences on Illness, 2nd ed. Tarzana, CA: Third Line Press, 354–355, 1009.

21. Nalder BN, et al. Sensitivity of the immunological response to the nutritional status of rats. *J Nutr* 102(4): 535–541, 1972. As cited in Werbach, p. 355.

22. Sanchez A, et al. Role of sugars in human neutrophilic phagocytosis. *Am J Clin Nutr* 26: 180, 1973. As cited in Werbach, p. 355.

23. Melamed I, et al. Coffee and the immune system. *Int J Immunol* 12: 129–134, 1990. As cited in Werbach, p. 355.

24. Kraal JH. Immunoglobulin levels in relation to smoking and coffee consumption. *Am J Clin Nutr* 31(2): 198–200, 1972. As cited in Werbach, p. 355.

Index

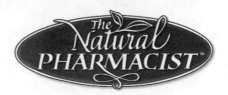

About the Author

Liz Collins, N.D., is a graduate of Reed College and the National College of Naturopathic Medicine. She practices family medicine and natural childbirth and also teaches at the National College of Naturopathic Medicine. Dr. Collins lives with her husband, David, in Portland, Oregon.

Nancy Berkoff, R.D., Ed.D., is a registered dietician, food technologist, and certified chef. She divides her time between teaching nutrition and culinary arts, food writing, and consulting.

About the Series Editors

Steven Bratman, M.D., medical director of Prima Health, has many years of experience in the alternative medicine field. A graduate of the University of California at Davis, Medical School, he has also trained in herbology, nutrition, Chinese medicine, and other alternative therapies, and has worked closely with a wide variety of alternative practitioners. He is the author of *The Natural Pharmacist: Your Complete Guide to Herbs* (Prima), *The Natural Pharmacist: Your Complete Guide to Illnesses and Their Natural Remedies* (Prima), *The Natural Pharmacist Guide to St. John's Wort and Depression* (Prima), *The Alternative Medicine Ratings Guide* (Prima), and *The Alternative Medicine Sourcebook* (Lowell House).

David J. Kroll, Ph.D., is a professor of pharmacology and toxicology at the University of Colorado School of Pharmacy and a consultant for pharmacists, physicians, and alternative practitioners on the indications and cautions for herbal medicine use. A graduate of both the University of Florida and the Philadelphia College of Pharmacy and Science, Dr. Kroll has lectured widely and has published articles in a number of medical journals, abstracts, and newsletters.